D0915409

Chronic Condition

Why Health Reform Fails

//////////

Sherry Glied

Harvard University Press

Cambridge, Massachusetts
London, England
1997

Library of Congress Cataloging-in-Publication Data

Glied, Sherry.
    Chronic condition : why health reform fails / Sherry Glied.
      p. cm.
    Includes bibliographical references and index.
    ISBN 0-674-12893-1 (alk. paper)
    1. Health care reform—Political aspects—United States.
    2. Health care reform—Economic aspects—United States.
    I. Title.
    RA395.A3G54   1997
    362.1'0973—dc21   97-23827

To my parents

Contents

Illustrations

Tables

Preface

From August 1992 through July 1993, I served as a senior economist for the president's Council of Economic Advisers. It was an auspicious time to be working on health issues in Washington. I had been recruited to help with the analysis of President George Bush's health plan. Then, in January 1993, with President Bill Clinton's inauguration, health reform moved to the center of the political stage. As one of the five hundred members of the president's health reform task force, I participated in the discussions about the design of the reform plan. As the council chair's health economics adviser, I also attended cabinet meetings and presidential briefings, where I had the unusual opportunity of seeing the reform design debates from the vantage point of the principal decision makers.

In the fall of 1993, I returned to Columbia University and gave seminars on health reform for my colleagues in the School of Public Health and the Department of Economics. They were nearly unanimous in their dissatisfaction with the Clinton health plan, but the reasons for unhappiness at the School of Public Health and in the economics department could hardly have been less similar. Where one group saw groveling to private-sector interests, the other saw massive public intervention and overregulation. Where one group saw a perpetuation of existing inequities, the other saw aggressive redistribution.

This book is my attempt to make sense of what I saw in Washington as well as what I heard in New York. I could not have written it had I not worked for the Council of Economic Advisers in Washington. The council is a wonderful institution that adds enormous value both to the government that employs it and to the economists who work for it. I am very grateful to Michael Boskin, the chair of the council when I was appointed, for giving me the chance to be one of those economists. Laura D'Andrea Tyson was council chair in the Clinton administration during my tenure. She encouraged the council's economists to attend and participate in high-level meetings, took our advice seriously, and gave us credit when she incorporated our analysis in her own arguments. It was an honor to work for her.

I learned a tremendous amount from the members of the council and the other senior and junior staff economists. I owe a special debt to David Bradford, who helped me wrestle with the logic of health economics while we wrote the 1993 Economic Report of the President and since; to David Cutler, who brought good sense, well-reasoned economics, and extraordinary energy to the health reform debate and provided useful comments on a draft of this book; and to Kim O'Neill Packard, who was an indispensable colleague throughout my time at the council.

I am also greatly indebted to those I worked with in Washington outside the council. My fellow members of the White House Task Force on Health Risk Pooling (especially Steve Bandeian and Jim Mays) equipped me with a thorough grounding in both the political and practical complications of health system reform. The health care task force provided a remarkable education in health policy. I am particularly appreciative of having worked with Judy Feder, Larry Levitt, Paul Starr, Marina Weiss, and Walter Zelman, as well as many of the other five hundred members.

Larry Brown painstakingly read and annotated an early draft of the manuscript. The book you are reading is much superior to the one he pored over, largely because of his questions and comments. Eli Ginzberg, Roz Lasker, and Bill Sage also read early versions of the book. Their suggestions led to valuable improvements and their enthusiasm provided timely encouragement. Joseph Newhouse and two anonymous reviewers for the Harvard University Press gave me very constructive criticisms that have made the book better. As with so much of my work, this book has benefited from discussions with David Bloom, an inimitable teacher and friend. It is only fair to note that none of those who worked with me or commented on my manuscript agree with me all of the time, and some of them disagree with me most of the time.

Michael Aronson encouraged me to write the book and shepherded (nudged?) me through the process of getting it completed, revised, accepted, and published. Michael Brandon ably edited it, Debojyoti

Sarkar helped with programming, Graphito produced the graphs, and Michelle Kofman and Sarah Wilson assisted with proofreading.

My husband, Richard Briffault, inspired me to write the book, spent countless hours listening to me prattle on about health reform, lovingly pointed out gaping holes in my logic, tracked down missing references, patiently polished my language through multiple drafts, and with good humor and affection maintained my equilibrium throughout the process. This project would have been unthinkable—and impossible—without him. Our daughter Olivia was born just as the book was accepted for publication, and she has joined her father in the work of keeping me cheerful through revisions and copyediting.

My mother's lifelong love, confidence, and support, confirmed daily in ways small and large, provided the foundation for this book and all my other endeavors. This is only the latest in a very long series of my compositions whose first reader has been my father. He is an ideal reader—uncompromising both in his expectations and in his belief that I can meet them. The book's style has profited from his specific comments. Its substance owes much to his often demonstrated conviction of the importance of uniting enterprise with compassion.

Chronic Condition

1 ///

Introduction

In the spring of 1993, comprehensive reform of the U.S. health care system seemed inevitable. In an April opinion poll, a majority of Americans asserted that even fundamental changes would not be enough to mend health care, and they called instead for a complete overhaul of the system. More than two-thirds of those polled favored a tax-financed national health insurance program (Jacobs, Shapiro, and Schulman 1993).

Republicans and Democrats, Congress and the White House—all seemed ready for significant action. Back in November of 1991, Pennsylvanian Harris Wofford, a political unknown campaigning on a platform of national health insurance, had climbed from forty points behind in the polls to beat former U.S. attorney general Richard Thornburgh in their race for a seat in the Senate. The stunning upset led to the introduction of more than seventy health reform bills in the following congressional session. While politicians disagreed about the best road to health reform, the primary goals of the effort—expanding coverage and reducing costs—were almost universally endorsed by members of Congress.

In February 1992, responding to the popular clamor for reform, President George Bush released a white paper proposing improvements in the health insurance system, changes in malpractice rules, and tax credits to enable poor Americans to buy insurance coverage. By the summer of 1992, Bill Clinton, campaigning for president, made health reform one of the centerpieces of his platform, calling for universal coverage financed through savings from a comprehensive cost-containment program. Three-quarters of voters ranked health care as a very important issue in the presidential campaign. On this issue the electorate favored Clinton over Bush almost three to one—an important difference in light of Clinton's narrow margin of victory. Finally, in September 1993, when President Clinton made his long-awaited health care speech to a joint session of Congress, it seemed as though universal health care coverage, a goal of reformers for more than five decades, was just around the corner. Clinton's speech was greeted by tumultuous applause, a conciliatory response from Senate Republican leader Bob Dole, and enthusiastic support from ordinary Americans.[1]

But now, in Clinton's second term, national health reform aimed at guaranteeing coverage to all Americans is a dead issue. Rather than expanding the government's role in the system, Congress is chipping away at existing federal programs, subordinating health care spending to the overarching goal of deficit reduction. Where members of Congress once confidently boasted of extending Medicare-like health coverage to all Americans, today they whisper about cutting benefits to those who already have public coverage. Rather than giving President Clinton and the Democratic party a boost in popular support, some pundits argued, the attempt to reform health care in fact contributed to the party's defeat in the 1994 midterm elections (Balz 1994). Even Harris Wofford, the man who brought health reform into the political limelight, lost his seat that November.

The spectacular failure of the Clinton administration's attempt at health reform cannot be blamed on the missteps of this particular administration. None of the alternative plans put forward by the right, the left, or the center ever garnered much support either. Nor did the demise of health reform occur because the system somehow cured itself. None of the things that bothered Americans about their health care system in 1993 disappeared of its own accord. Nor is it likely that health reform has fallen off the public agenda forever. While renewed skepticism about the ability of government to address health care concerns may undermine popular support for reform, the continuing pressures of rising Medicare and Medicaid program costs ensure that Congress cannot simply avoid the issue.

Unfortunately, as I argue in the remainder of this book, the health care reform proposals most often considered cannot solve the problems of the health care system. They may lead to short-term improvements and even to some budget savings, but over time they will undoubtedly fail. In this context, the downfall of the Clinton plan is not only a matter of historical interest. The failure of the plan stems from problems that plague all health reform plans. Indeed, some of the same obstacles stymied congressional efforts to reform the Medicare program.

Why Did Americans Want Health Reform?

Four issues drove health reform in the early 1990s: health security for the middle class, coverage for the uninsured, the mushrooming national cost of health care, and the effects of health spending on the federal budget.

Health Security

President Clinton called his plan for health care reform the Health Security Act. That title both alluded to the Social Security Act—President Franklin D. Roosevelt's popular legacy—and addressed a concern specific to health care. Even well-insured middle-class people fear that if they become ill or develop a marker for future illness, they will not be able to purchase health insurance coverage at affordable rates. Insurers today price policies according to the health condition of those who purchase them, and they often exclude preexisting health conditions from coverage.[2] For employees with good coverage through their current job, the risk of losing coverage is a disincentive to switching to a better job. Responding to these concerns, a central theme of the Health Security Act was to guarantee Americans benefits that could "never be taken away" (*Health Security Act* 1993).

To the president, and to many other policymakers, health security meant more than reform of the insurance market to constrain the extent of pricing according to health risk. Limiting risk-based pricing would lower the premiums of people with existing illnesses, but without further steps it would raise the premiums of Americans who were not ill. Such reforms might actually lead many young, healthy Americans to stop purchasing insurance coverage altogether. Furthermore, reform of the insurance market alone would not deliver coverage to most already uninsured Americans, and it would not erase the fear that losing a job might lead to a loss of health insurance coverage. Health security for the middle class would require more than simply improved coverage for the middle class. It would require universal coverage.

Coverage for the Uninsured

In the spring of 1993, more than 40 million Americans—15 percent of the population—lacked health insurance. The number of uninsured Americans had risen continuously every year since 1988 (see Figure 1.1).[3]

Being uninsured means getting less medical care. Although the uninsured do receive care, they receive substantially more limited care than do those with coverage; and the uninsured often receive medical attention later in the course of an illness, when doctors can do less to help them. Those who lack insurance may put off routine care. When they become seriously ill, most cannot, and do not, pay the cost of the

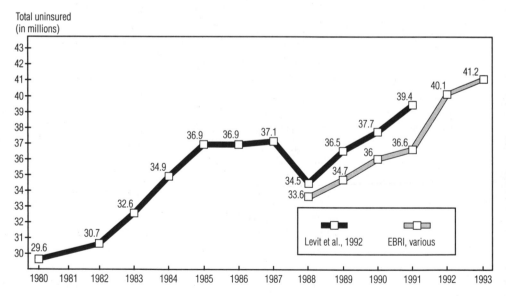

Figure 1.1 Estimates of the number of uninsured Americans, 1980–1993 (*Sources:* Levit, Olin, and Letsch 1992; EBRI various).

expensive care they receive. Instead, most of these costs are absorbed by government programs and the hospitals and doctors who provide care, who then attempt to pass the costs along to paying patients.

When asked, Americans express concern for the plight of the uninsured. Most believe the uninsured should be able to obtain appropriate health care, and many are willing to pay at least some additional taxes to finance the costs of this care.[4] An overwhelming majority believe that the poor should be entitled to health care as good as the rich receive. Americans recognize that in today's high-cost health care system, "poor people [cannot] receive needed care" (Jacobs, Shapiro, and Schulman 1993, p. 404).

Cost Containment

Health care in the United States today is very costly. Americans on average spend more than $3,300 a year per person on health care, 14 percent of the nation's income (Levit et al. 1994). Twice as much is spent on health care as on education, and about three times as much as on national defense. The United States spends about one-and-a-half times as much on care per capita as does Canada, the second-most-costly country. As Figure 1.2 shows, health care costs are projected to continue rising well into the future, consuming ever more of the nation's gross domestic product (GDP).

Americans, even those who can readily afford their own insurance and direct medical care costs, want to control those costs. In the spring of 1993, 84 percent favored directly limiting health spending and constraining costs to the growth of the national economy (Jacobs, Shapiro, and Schulman 1993). In the speech presenting his health plan to Congress, President Clinton argued that "our competitiveness, our whole economy, the integrity of the way our government works, and, ultimately, our living standards depend upon our ability to achieve savings without harming the quality of health care" (quoted in Drew 1994, p. 302).

Federal Budget Deficit

Even without universal coverage, existing federal health care programs have a sizable impact on the nation's budget—and on the budget def-

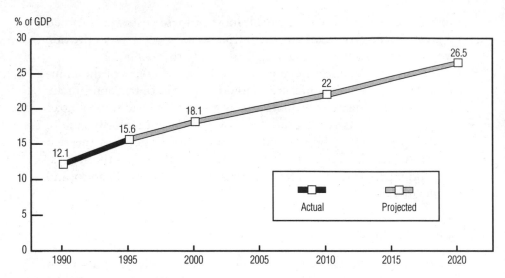

Figure 1.2 Health care as a share of U.S. GDP, 1990–2020 (projected). (*Source:* Burner, Waldo, and McKusick 1992.)

icit. Medicare and Medicaid, the largest federal health programs, cost $275 billion in fiscal year 1995 and have been growing at a rate of 10 to 13 percent a year (CBO 1994a). Growing federal health care spending has subverted efforts to control the deficit. In President Clinton's first budget, delivered to Congress before the health plan had been formulated, almost 60 percent of new spending went to health programs. Projections show this problem getting worse. By 2000 over one-quarter of the federal budget will be devoted to health care. State and local governments also chafe under the increased burden of health spending. By the turn of the century states may be spending as much of their budgets on health care as they do on elementary and secondary education today.

The four problems of security, coverage of the uninsured, cost, and the budget are interrelated. If coverage were universal, security wouldn't be a problem. If health care didn't cost so much, it wouldn't be so hard to cover the uninsured. If existing federal programs didn't cost so much, it would be easier for the government to subsidize more people. Piecemeal reform can exacerbate one problem while curing another.

The advantage of comprehensive reform is that it provides an opportunity to solve the whole health care puzzle at once.

President Clinton's Proposal

Before taking office in January 1993, President Clinton promised the American people that he would bring them a plan for reform of the health system within 100 days of the inauguration. He missed the deadline by about 100 days, but in September and October 1993 he presented first a speech and then a plan for reform to Congress.

President Clinton's plan combined elements from two well-known policy proposals: single payer and managed competition. Under the single-payer concept, the government would assure health coverage to all. The government would pay all health bills, compensating doctors, hospitals, and other health providers according to centrally established fee schedules. By adjusting fee schedules (and taking other regulatory actions), the government would control the total amount the country spent on health care.

The second plan, managed competition, envisions a system of competing private insurers operating in a government-regulated marketplace. The managed-competition proposal emphasizes the importance of giving both consumers, who buy health care, and health care professionals, who provide care, incentives to use resources in the most cost-effective ways.

Academic researchers, interest groups, and policymakers have spent the past two decades refining these reform designs into coherent proposals. At the beginning of the decade, though, neither plan had the support of a majority of policymakers. In response to perceived failings in each of these plans, a small group of health policy analysts forged a new, compromise plan that they called managed competition under a budget.[5] This compromise plan, which combined the government-established limits on spending characteristic of the single-payer plan with the incentive-oriented competition among health plans that marked the managed-competition plan, became the basis for President Clinton's reform effort.

President Clinton's proposal, the Health Security Act, blended elements from existing plans and directly addressed each of the concerns that motivated the interest in health reform. Insurers would not be permitted to charge more to those with health problems and could not limit coverage for preexisting conditions, so under the plan, those in ill health would no longer pay higher insurance premiums. Consumers, rather than their employers, would choose their own health plans so that the fears of losing or being forced to change insurance as a consequence of a job change would be eliminated.

The plan would provide universal coverage. An employer mandate would ensure that all working Americans could participate in the system. Those not working would also be required to participate, and a system of government subsidies would help them afford coverage. All insurers would cover the same benefits and meet the same quality standards. Regulations would ensure that the quality of care received by poor Americans would not fall substantially below that received by those with higher incomes.

Both the regulatory and incentive-oriented elements of the plan would work to rein in costs. Consumers would have substantial incentives to seek lower-cost plans. In case these incentives did not keep costs in check, the plan included a cap on premium increases to ensure that costs did not increase faster than national income.

Finally, the plan would help the government balance the federal budget. Most of the financing would come through the employer mandate and flow directly to health insurers without ever passing through Washington. The cap on premiums, translated into limits on the growth of existing health programs, would reduce the rate of growth in federal health costs. Federal subsidies for low-wage employers and low-income Americans would not be allowed to grow any faster than the premium cap.

Why Did the Plan Fail?

On the surface, the Health Security Act seemed to solve every major problem propelling the interest in national health reform. It addressed the concerns of the uninsured and those who worried about becoming uninsured, and it guaranteed cost containment for the nation as a whole and for the government. It creatively combined elements from two of the most popular reform plans. Why then did it fail?

Supporters of health reform contend that politics doomed the Health

Security Act. While political factors were extremely important, they alone cannot account for the failure of the effort. Rather, the failure of the plan stemmed from the three problems that are the focus of most of this book. First, the beliefs that shape the proposals of the two main groups of reformers—those who support single-payer reform and those who support a more market-oriented, managed-competition approach—are so different that compromise is impossible. Second, both groups base their policy prescriptions on false assumptions about health care spending and the health sector, so their proposals are undermined as the weakness of their assumptions comes to light. Third, neither group successfully addresses the financing of health care reform. In today's antitax climate, both groups do whatever they can to avoid mentioning the fact that health reform must either cost money or reduce health care use.

Political Failures

There is no doubt that a variety of political factors severely handicapped the Clinton administration's efforts at health reform. But before analyzing the failure of current health policy initiatives, I want to make the case that the alternative hypotheses for why the Clinton plan failed—the strength of health care lobbies, the strategic ineptness of the administration, the complexity of the plan itself, the employer-mandate financing system, partisan politics—are not sufficient to explain the collapse of reform.

The death of past health reform efforts has been ascribed to opposition from health care interest groups.[6] The American Medical Association (AMA), the leading representative of doctors, almost scotched Medicare by railing about the dangers of socialized medicine. Health care lobbyists certainly participated actively in the 1993 debate and made substantial contributions to the political campaigns of both Democrats and Republicans. The health insurance industry, mounting a direct attack on the plan, ran a series of ads highly critical of the Clinton proposal.

Health lobbyists made it harder to pass the Clinton plan, but it is important not to overstate their role. Both the American Medical Association and the Health Insurance Association of America supported universal coverage and the requirement that employers pay part of health care bills (Starr 1995). In the wake of years of declining health insurance coverage, both groups had self-interested reasons for wanting some kind of health reform to pass. Most of the health care interest groups lobbied not against the passage of any legislation but for modifications of legislation to serve their own interests. Lobbying efforts did jeopardize particular features of the Clinton plan, but they did not turn the political climate against reform altogether.

Some observers of the political process have blamed the failure of the Health Security Act on political bungling by the Clinton administration. A number complain that Clinton's reform plan was designed in secrecy by a shadowy health care task force rather than in an open, public process. Others argue that the administration was too open to the complaints of outside interest groups and too quick to compromise. Some assert that the president seemed too ready to negotiate with Congress; others believe that he should have allowed the legislators to develop a plan themselves.[7] While more savvy political tactics would have helped the president, they do not explain the failure of the congressional efforts to develop a plan. By the fall of 1994, the president's plan was dead—but so were plans developed by representatives and senators well versed in political strategy.

The complexity of the Clinton plan, critics say, provides ample illustration of the political naïveté of its designers. The managed-competition structure depended on the creation of a hierarchy of new institutions—ready ammunition for analysts on the left and right who decried the construction of a brand-new bureaucracy. Combining these elements with the enforcement and monitoring structures needed to ensure compliance with the premium cap yielded a plan so mazelike that only a few hardy analysts could hope to negotiate it.[8]

The administration could and probably should have made the plan simpler by excluding peripheral elements, such as legislation to improve the Indian Health Service, reform medical education, improve Medicare's long-term-care coverage, and tie the health insurance system to the workers' compensation system. The elaborate structure of the plan, though, was largely a necessary consequence of its attempt to combine the managed-competition and single-payer proposals. The administration needed to guarantee that it could produce savings while providing universal and equitable coverage and retaining a market-based health insurance system. The difficulties of balancing all three objectives became evident as alternative "centrist" plans advanced in the House and Senate. Plans that relied on private insurance inevitably faltered when they had to guarantee to budget hawks that savings could be achieved.

Finally, the administration faced furious opposition from small-business interests angered by the employer-mandate financing system. In fact, the subsidy structure in the administration's plan provided substantial advantages to small businesses.[9] The smallest, lowest-wage businesses would pay only 3.5 percent of payroll for health insurance coverage, the equivalent of a 15-cent increase in the minimum wage. In polls most Americans supported requiring employers to purchase coverage for their employees. Nonetheless, the administration never effectively countered the small-business attack. Here, too, though, the peculiarities of the administration's plan cannot be blamed for the failure of the entire health reform effort. The administration and congressional reformers considered a panoply of alternative financing sources for health reform, from broad-based taxes to individual mandates. These plans, too, were swept away as the tide turned against health reform.

By the end of the process, congressional Republicans, some of whom had originally supported reform and even proposed reform bills of their own, recognized the partisan advantages of thwarting the president's initiative altogether. Senate minority leader Dole, who had originally applauded the president's efforts, now moved away from even his own earlier, moderate reform plan. Partisan politics was the proximate cause of the downfall of the Clinton reform proposal. But the nature of partisan politicking around the plan was itself a consequence of the general lack of enthusiasm for the plan. Republicans swung away from the plan only when it failed to garner widespread support.

Failure to Compromise

For those in the administration who designed the reform plans, the most disheartening aspect of the health reform debate was the tepid support offered by longtime partisans of health reform—the liberal lobbying groups, big businesses, unions, and assorted academics who had insisted that reform was essential. The Clinton plan was, after all, intended as a compromise between the two major camps of health reformers: those who favored a single-payer system and those who favored managed competition. Although no one expects a compromise to garner enormous enthusiasm, administration officials did expect that their proposal would form the basis for negotiation. That did not happen. Instead, the only thing both camps agreed to do was to dismantle the health alliances, the structural linchpin of the Clinton plan.

Differences among groups pressing for reform were a key factor in the deadlock on structural change. These differences stem from the distinct and conflicting views of health care held by the two main groups of reformers. Supporters of the single-payer plan do not just believe that their plan provides the best technical solution to the problems of the health care system. They also believe that medical care is quite different from other goods and services; that doctors, not consumers, should and do make health care decisions; that markets are an inappropriate instrument for allocating health care; and that health care should be distributed in an egalitarian fashion. Managed-competition supporters, by contrast, view health care as a good much like other goods. They grant preeminence to consumer choices, favor markets over bureaucracy, and would accept a less equal distribution of health care. In the discussion of these views in Chapter 2, I refer to the views of single-payer supporters as "medicalist" views and to the views of managed-competition supporters as "marketist" views.

The proposals advanced by the two groups share goals and themes. Advocates of both styles of reform complain of massive inefficiency and waste in the current system. Each group maintains that its reform proposal could save enough money to expand coverage substantially without rationing care or raising taxes. Yet despite the rhetorical similarities between proponents of the two views and despite their agreement on the need for and goals of reform, their fundamental philosophies concerning the nature of health care and the role of markets are profoundly antithetical and deeply resistant to compromise.

Any significant reform of the health care system would entrench the views of one or the other group. As each side fought hard to avoid losing the battle over the future of health policy, it rejected proposals that would make any structural changes to the existing system that did not incorporate its basic assumptions. The only politically viable reforms that remain are modest adjustments to the existing institutional structure. The failure of structural health reform can be blamed as much on those who favored reform as on those who opposed it.

What Next?

For a policymaker, whether a medicalist or a marketist, health care certainly *is* different from other policy-relevant goods and services. Other policy problems can be addressed once every twenty or thirty years; health reform never seems to go away. Health care changes constantly and rapidly. Consumers, who experience the pain and misery of illness and disability, quite sensibly demand more and more of this ever improving product. Costs, equally inexorably, rise. Policymakers must refinance or revamp their existing programs and address the concerns of those who now can no longer afford insurance coverage. By the time they finish acting, health care has changed again, setting off another cycle of policy action.

There is nothing new about this problem. Health care spending has been rising quite steadily since 1935, as Figure 1.3 shows. Figure 1.3 plots per capita spending (adjusted for economy-wide inflation) on a logarithmic scale. A straight line on a logarithmic scale, like the plot of health spending after 1935, implies that costs have been growing at a constant rate. Per capita health costs in the United States have grown at an average annual inflation-adjusted rate of 4 to 5 percent since 1935. This simple reality has two profound implications. First, as I show in Chapter 3, the potential money savings from any commonly cited reform of the system—such as administrative simplification, malpractice reform, or higher consumer out-of-pocket payments—pale in comparison with the differences in health spending from one year to the next. At best, reducing waste and inefficiencies today could free up resources for covering today's costs of caring for the poor and uninsured. But it would fail to cover the uninsured tomorrow, as costs continue to rise. Second—and more important, given the dynamic nature of health care—health reform proposals should be judged according to how well they respond to the problems of the future, not those of today. As I explain, neither of the two camps of health reformers proposes policy prescriptions that contend with the future of health care.

Medicalists support a government-run system that is centrally organized and financed. Such a system could produce egalitarian universal coverage along with health security for all, forever—but at a considerable price. A government-run, centrally organized system would re-

Log of per capita health spending

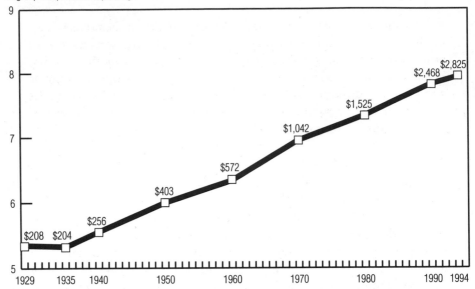

Figure 1.3 The growth of health spending in the United States, 1929–1994. Per capita expenditures are depicted in constant (1991) dollars on a log scale. (*Sources:* 1929–1960 from Department of Commerce, 1975; 1961–1990 from Letsch et al. 1992; 1991–1994 from U.S. Department of Health and Human Services Web Site.)

tard organizational innovation. It would respond more slowly and less flexibly to inevitable, desirable changes in health care technology and consumer preferences. Such a system is at odds with the evolving nature of health care. Moreover, financing health care centrally means balancing the benefits of improved health technologies against the political and economic cost of higher taxes. The experiences of the Canadian health system and of the Medicare program show that this balancing act imposes an enormous strain on public finances. In time it leads to cutbacks in health spending that impose costs in terms of discomfort, inconvenience, and uncertainty that at least some citizens would gladly pay to avoid. As I discuss in Chapter 4, by making life—and medical treatment—more comfortable and less inconvenient, rising health care spending has almost certainly improved, rather than harmed, America's national well-being. Constraining health spending to some predetermined fraction of national income would make some people worse off.

Rising health expenditures in aggregate make life better, but in the current U.S. health care system, some groups bear much more of the burden of rising expenditures than do others. In Chapter 5 I examine the problems of redistributing health care resources. Medicalists would limit increases in expenditures by slowing organizational and technological change in health care. While these restraints can reduce the quality of care, they also simplify the problems associated with distributing resources. Once a redistribution scheme is in place, technological and organizational change will occur slowly, allowing the process for financing health care to operate indefinitely.[10]

The competitive system supported by marketists avoids many of the problems of regulatory intervention and limits the fiscal vulnerability of the national treasury that plagues medicalist solutions. But the market solution has difficulty addressing the distributional concerns of health reformers. Market-based reform cannot promise adequate universal coverage and health security as health care changes. Marketists would permit rapid technological and organizational innovation, but would offer financing only for some predetermined and static "adequate" level of care. Americans' view of adequate care for others changes along with their view of adequate care for themselves. The marketist model, though, provides no way of judging how much should be spent to meet the changing costs of health care for those who cannot pay their own medical bills and have no way of financing these ever increasing costs.

Medicalists and marketists turn their particular views of health care into plans for reform by developing particular institutional models, such as the single-payer model and the managed-competition model. To be successful these institutional structures must accommodate changes in health care that improve people's well-being. As I indicate in Chapter 6, the plans advanced by both medicalists and marketists fail this test in important ways. Medicalists rely heavily on a regulatory process that is likely to react slowly to change and to favor the interests of well-organized advocacy groups over the routine demands of ordinary Americans. Marketists criticize the regulatory process but fail to devote much attention to the less pervasive, yet nonetheless important, institutional structures of their own reform plans.

The weaknesses of both medicalist and marketist approaches suggest that reform along either line is unlikely to work in the long term. The appeal of a compromise solution, embraced by the Clinton administration, was to move away from these ideologically polarized visions of health care to a technical solution that drew on the strengths of the institutional structures developed by both models. But the fundamental logical conflict between the two plans means that true compromise is impossible.

Instead, the plan the administration finally developed was not so much a synthesis of the two plans as a concatenation of a marketist and a medicalist model: not managed competition under a budget, but managed competition that would turn into a budget. If costs did not rise, markets, albeit heavily regulated ones, would be used to finance and distribute health care. If costs did rise, an alternative, heavily regulatory institutional structure would manage the system. As I discuss in Chapter 7, the decision to adopt this two-part plan arose as a way of mediating between the two models, but its final form was dictated by the strictures of the federal budget deficit. The federal budget deficit also undermined Congress's effort to legislate a purely marketist reform of the federal Medicare program in 1995.

The future of health care in America cannot be resolved by either the medicalist or the marketist policies that have been advanced so far. The egalitarian structure of medicalist models will erode as governments cut back services in the face of rising costs and stagnant revenues. The competitive processes on which marketists rely will be undermined as politicians strive to keep down the cost of care funded through government programs. In Chapter 8 I propose a direct tax on health care spending. This method of financing reform is consistent with either a marketist or a medicalist approach and would move the United States in the direction of a more sustainable system. In the context of marketist reform, this proposal would allow individual health care choices to yield an appropriate level of national health spending. At the same time, my proposal would provide a means of funding and redistributing health resources that would maintain a constantly changing "adequate" standard of care for all Americans.

2 ///

Medicalists and Marketists

Active participants in the U.S. health reform debate adhere to two very different sets of views about the nature of health care—as a market "good" or a medically determined "need." The political debate between supporters of Canadian-style single-payer reforms and market-competition-oriented models of reform reflects this underlying conflict about how even to think about health care. Deep differences in basic assumptions fuel the policy battles over such issues as how to control the cost of health care and what institutional structure reform should adopt. In this chapter I describe and critique the basic tenets of these views and focus on the ways their proponents approach the problems inherent in providing care to the poor and confronting rapidly changing health care technologies.

Marketists

The view that health care is a market good—the approach I call the marketist perspective on health care—emerges from neoclassical economics. Not all neoclassical economists are marketists and not all marketists are economists. Indeed, some of the most important articles in health economics make the case that the market does not work properly in health care (Arrow 1963; Evans 1974). Nonetheless, because the central belief of adherents of this approach to health reform is that the market is the best way to allocate health care, the term *marketist* is appropriate.[1]

Marketists see health care as just another good or service, not in any fundamental way different from "other commodities bought and sold on the open market" (Burns 1973, p. 25), and, like all other goods and services, best allocated through the market. In this view consumers choose to purchase health care services when the value to them of a unit of these services exceeds (or equals) its cost to them. Marketists argue that "there is no better basis for judging the value of a [health] service than the willingness of a person to pay for that service" (Pauly et al. 1992, p. 50). The value of health services, then, depends critically on the consumer's idiosyncratic preferences, income, and other opportunities. In turn, producers provide health care services up to the point at which their price equals the cost of producing them.

Markets for most goods and services other than health care operate more or less efficiently, in the economists' sense that they produce the goods and services that consumers most prize at the lowest attainable cost. What makes health care today different from these other goods, in the marketists' view, is that the government plays an enormous role in the health care market. Federal and state governments together pay 45 percent of U.S. health bills (CBO 1992). Including the $79 billion cost associated with the government's preferential tax treatment for employer-provided private health insurance, the U.S. government pays for a larger share of the output of the health care sector than it does of the defense-dominated aerospace sector (CEA 1993; Glied 1994). There are more government-employed health and hospital workers as than there are postal workers (CEA 1993).

Marketists argue that the government distorts the demand for health care, particularly by excluding from income and payroll taxation the value of employer-provided health insurance. This distortion is viewed by marketists as the principal source of correctable inefficiency in the health care market (Feldstein 1977; Pauly 1986). The substantial benefits of this favorable tax treatment encourage policyholders to buy coverage for services that carry little financial risk and to resist features of health insurance policies that would limit overuse of services. More radical—or less diplomatic—marketists complain equally about the distortions induced by the Medicare program. Medicare, which covers elderly and disabled Americans, is a centrally regulated program that leaves little scope for market pricing. Prices are set centrally, so Medicare beneficiaries have no opportunity to benefit from choosing lower-cost providers. Most beneficiaries purchase government-sanctioned supplemental coverage that leaves them with little incentive to seek lower-cost care.

The supply of health care services is also complicated by government-induced distortions. Foremost among these is the government-sanctioned self-regulating power of American physicians. Physicians, through state-established licensing boards, decide how many new entrants may join the profession. They have used this power to keep earnings above competitive levels and to slow the development of new forms of insurance and physician payment (Kessel 1958; Starr 1982). According to marketists, other regulatory interventions in the market, such as certificate-of-need regulations intended to rationalize the distribution of hospital beds and high-technology equipment, similarly favor the interests of those being regulated. Regulations increase costs by perpetuating existing hospitals and foreclosing entry by less costly competitors (Feldstein 1988).

The view of health care as just another good has strong implications for both the best method of organizing the health system and the preferred distribution of health resources. From an allocative perspective, the key problem for marketists is ensuring that "the price is right." In neoclassical economic theory, if consumers and producers face prices that reflect the underlying costs of production and the intensity of consumer preferences, the economy will operate efficiently, producing the most highly valued goods and services at the lowest prices and distributing them to those consumers who most value them.

A related explanation of why proper pricing matters draws on the economic theories of Friederich Hayek. In Hayek's view, getting prices right is important because prices provide the most rapid means of conveying information to producers and consumers. Prices are especially critical in health care because of the swiftly changing and complex nature of health care service provision (Hayek 1945). Health care service provision today involves multiple producers (doctors, hospital, drug companies) and multiple strategies of production (bed rest, inpatient surgery, outpatient surgery, pharmaceutical treatment). Prices tell buyers and sellers the relative costliness and effectiveness of these alternative courses of treatment. When new technologies are developed, prices throughout the market adjust, encouraging producers to abandon obsolete methods of treatment and adopt better ones.

In health care, price-prompted change often takes the form of changes in the nature of health care organizations. Health care has experienced twenty years of rapid organizational innovation. Health maintenance organizations (HMOs) and preferred provider organizations (PPOs), in which insurers contract with a limited number of doctors and hospitals to create a vertically integrated delivery system, have captured over half of the health care market (Weiner and de Lissovoy 1993; CEA 1995). New firms have entered the market providing specialized oversight services (utilization management) to conventional insurers. Accreditation organizations, dedicated to overseeing the qualifications of utilization reviewers and of vertically integrated health providers, have arisen in response to these innovations. Marketists view the proliferation of these organizations as a natural response to rapid changes in health technologies.[2] As new techniques, products, and providers are introduced, payers must assess their quality and efficacy and decide how to pay for them. Vertical integration and specialized oversight can help address these problems.

The marketist model of health care (like economic approaches generally) emphasizes efficiency issues. Proponents of this model do not view the cost of health care, in itself, as a matter of concern. They argue that "consumers' choices will, by definition, lead to the right rate of growth of cost" (Pauly et al. 1992, p. 47). Health care as a share of GDP is irrelevant in a model in which consumers freely express their preferences by buying care. Rather, government-induced market distortions lead to inefficiency in the system. The existence of inefficiency implies that resources are wasted, and it is in this sense that costs must be contained. Wasted costs, but only wasted costs, must be contained. Costs that are due to informed consumer choices are no cause for concern.

The Marketist Model and the Poor

In the pure marketist model, the cost of care (an efficiency issue) can be divorced from the question of the redistribution of care (an equity issue). In the marketist view, society needs to decide how much money to spend on the poor. At that point the distributional question with respect to health care is best addressed the way all distributional questions ought to be addressed: by redistributing income. Marketists see no point to subsidizing health care itself. Once the poor have income, they can maximize utility by choosing health care or other goods and services according to their own preferences.

Redistribution, in the marketist model, has undesirable side effects, particularly when it is based on criteria other than low income. Redistributing health care to the sick, for example, provides poor health incentives. So much of health care depends on what we do for ourselves, and redistribution tied to health status reduces the value of taking care (Roberts 1986). Smokers, speeders, steak fanciers, and the sedentary increase their own risks of poor health. Forcing the health-conscious to subsidize risk takers only weakens the nation's health. Redistributing care on the basis of age gives middle-aged people less incentive to save for retirement. It may even weaken the bonds between parents and children as parents no longer need to depend on their children to care for them in their old age (Frum 1994).

Marketists prefer income redistribution, but they find even this kind of redistribution fraught with difficulties. Taxing those with high incomes gives them disincentives to work; providing services to the poor reduces their incentive to improve their state. Taxing labor reduces employment; taxing capital reduces growth. While the marketist model recognizes the call for redistribution, it finds the reality problematic.

The institutional structure favored by marketists emphasizes removing existing distortions in the health market such as the favorable tax treatment of health insurance. Marketists would limit the government's role to the least intrusive redistributive mechanism feasible. Once redistribution has been accomplished, marketist reformers expect private, competing insurers to solve allocation problems in the modern health marketplace. Insurers protect people against the financial risk of unanticipated illness, leaving consumers with sufficient incentives to make appropriately cost-conscious choices about their care. As "managed care" companies, insurers can offer consumers a package deal (a premium) for a set of potentially necessary services (a benefit package). In this guise, they also act as allocation experts, combining services to offer the most cost-effective treatment for a given condition.

Critiques of the Marketist Model

The first line of attack on the market model comes from economists who argue that health care lacks the features that distinguish goods and services that can be efficiently traded in an unregulated market. A well-functioning market requires well-informed consumers. But health care consumers have little information with which to judge the quality of the care they receive (Arrow 1963). Consumers may willingly pay the high prices charged by their providers for health care services or purchase low-quality services at discount prices because they are ignorant of the true costs and benefits of these procedures. In this environment market-driven insurers, providers, and managed-care companies may harm their uninformed customers.

Marketists counter that a variety of market institutions bridge the knowledge gap between patients and providers. Consumers use family doctors, whose quality they can presumably recognize, as advisers to help them negotiate the hospital and specialist markets (Pauly 1988). In recent years private and public efforts to improve the quality of consumer information in medicine have also progressed rapidly (CEA 1993). The growing use of managed care and similar arrangements where insurers contract directly with physicians may actually improve the prospects for consumers to make sensible quality choices. Insurers and managed-care organizations, like airlines and auto manufacturers, develop credible reputations for quality and thus simplify the consumer's choice problem (Klein and Leffler 1981; Getzen 1984). Health plans, consisting of large numbers of investors and physicians whose earnings depend on the reputation of the plan and who, in some cases, may be at direct financial risk if a member physician acts negligently, may well implement more safeguards to protect patient interests than would independent, private physicians (Carr and Mathewson 1990; Svorny 1992). Finally, marketists argue, the tort litigation system can be exploited to impose appropriate penalties against malicious or negligent providers (White 1994).

Marketists argue that this information asymmetry argument is somewhat disingenuous as a criticism of market-based reform. A lack of consumer information, in itself, does not distinguish health care from most other professional services. Consumers regularly employ brokers to help them pick stocks, lawyers to help them write contracts, real-estate agents to help them sell their homes, and accountants to help them comply with the tax laws. Informational asymmetries that lead uninformed consumers to hire highly trained experts explain the very existence of these apparently well-functioning professional-services markets.

The second important source of deviation from the standard economic framework of a perfectly functioning market arises because of the pervasiveness of insurance in the health care market. Almost 75 percent of American health bills are paid by third parties, not by the patient who incurs the expense (CBO 1993c). Well-insured patients may not make choices with appropriate regard for the cost of their care. Furthermore, economic theory suggests that if consumers can assess their own health status and choose their own plans, a competitive insurance market can disintegrate. Low-risk consumers will leave the market, driving up prices for those who remain, until no one buys coverage at all.

Marketists assert that the health insurance market has developed a number of successful responses to the problem of overutilization of services by the insured. Health insurance plans have a variety of mechanisms available to limit patients' use of services. Consumers can choose from an array of plans offering every imaginable permutation, from traditional insurance (where consumers pay a substantial share of costs through high deductible and coinsurance rates) to clinic-based health maintenance organization care (with insurer oversight of all care decisions) and virtually all points in between. While government policy may bias choices away from utilization control, the mechanisms for such control within the private insurance market undoubtedly exist. Health insurance customers today can hire their own regulator (Pauly 1988).

Institutional responses also appear to have largely overcome the problem of low-risk consumers leaving the health insurance market altogether. The widespread use of preexisting-condition clauses in insurance contracts makes the option of remaining uninsured until a catastrophe occurs relatively unattractive (Gabel et al. 1994). The prevalence of employer-based insurance also limits the opportunities for entering and leaving the market according to health status. Insurance pricing practices suggest that consumers can withhold relatively little information from insurers when making their purchasing choice.

Insurance is pervasive in modern economies and flourishes in many contexts in which consumer behavior both before and after the purchase of coverage seems more important than in the health market. Fashion models insure their hands; producers of horror movies about killer bees insure against the risk of bee stings; computer manufacturers insure against the risk that they inadvertently infringe on another firm's patent; chemical producers insure against hazardous-waste spills; and so on. Insurance does not appear to inhibit the functioning of these other sectors. Marketists argue that the dangers associated with a competitive insurance market have been vastly overstated.

History supports the argument that insurance by itself does not explain the problems of the health insurance market. The high cost and inefficiency of the system was a source of complaint in the 1920s, well before the introduction of widespread public or commercial health insurance in the United States (Starr 1982). The movement toward a formal public role in health coverage also predates the introduction of commercial insurance. Bismarck introduced sickness insurance in Germany by 1883, half a century before the formation of Blue Cross in the United States.

Marketists and the Changing Nature of Medical Care

The greatest flaw in the market model (as I discuss in more detail in Chapter 5) is its treatment of redistribution. U.S. health policy has often operated quite differently from the model envisioned by either the marketists or their economist critics. Reformers, and much of the public, worry more about the underuse of services by the uninsured than about the overuse of services by those with generous coverage. They worry more about the inability of those who are already ill to obtain coverage than about any propensity of the healthy to shun coverage. Americans, notoriously stingy about redistributing income, regularly provide extremely costly medical interventions to the indigent.

These concerns and behaviors fit poorly into the pure marketist model, which views redistribution in health care as simply a special case of income redistribution (Roberts 1986). They fit clumsily, as well, into an augmented marketist model that proposes, in lieu of income redistribution, that all Americans be assured of an "adequate" level of health coverage. As earlier commentators noted, "when Americans speak of 'adequate medical care,' they do not have in mind any finite or defined quantity or quality. The very concept is in a continuous state of flux with what is being achieved and is generally thought to be available" (Somers and Somers 1961, p. 138). The marketists' focus on the decisions of individuals neglects a critical feature of health care. Spending decisions related to health care encompass more than individual transactions. The availability of health resources, primarily determined by the spending decisions of the nonpoor, affects our expectations about the appropriate level of care offered to those who cannot afford to purchase care for themselves. Health care spending appears to be affected by the health care environment, not just each individual's income, preferences, and health status.

Interrelationships between people's health care choices have important implications for health policy, especially for policies that extend care to the poor. Health care is different from other goods and services in the way it is provided to the poor. Health care in the United States is certainly not distributed equitably today, but the poor receive more equitable treatment with respect to health care than with respect to most other goods. Federal and state programs directly provide health insurance and care to more than 23 million Americans who are under the age of sixty-five and whose income is below 200 percent of the poverty line (EBRI 1993). These programs are supplemented by a regulatory safety net. Most U.S. hospitals are required to admit and care for indigent patients who require emergency services. In 1991 private hospitals in the United States provided more than $13 billion in care for patients who could not pay directly (CBO 1993c),[3] and analysts suggest that as much as 10 percent of the care provided by American physicians is uncompensated (Kilpatrick et al. 1991). Americans supplement tax-paid programs with substantial charitable donations to health providers—more than $10 billion in 1981 (Andreoni 1988). Paradoxically, while the uninsured may not be able to afford routine care, they can often get complicated high-technology treatments if they become sick enough (Weissman and Epstein 1994).

The special treatment of the poor with respect to health care has complex effects in an environment of rapidly changing technology. When people who are not poor choose to use a new procedure, that revises the definition of "adequate medical care." In turn, that procedure is often also provided to the poor. The existence of the procedure means that the range of services provided to those who cannot pay for care expands.

The straightforward income-based redistribution programs envisioned by marketists fail to take this pattern into account. Unfortunately, it is very hard to graft more elaborate redistributive schemes onto market models. The minimalist institutional framework envisioned by marketists cannot withstand the weight of intricate redistributional mechanisms. By inclination marketists think about markets and disdain the bureaucracies that would be necessary to implement more elaborate schemes.

Medicalists

Many policymakers and most members of the public reject the marketist view of health care as just another commodity. Individual preferences determine the demand for most goods and services, but health care, as one writer memorably put it, is not "tomatoes" (Vladeck 1981). There is a "deep-seated belief . . . that medical care is not a commodity, that its characteristics are scientifically determined, and that decisions concerning it must be entrusted exclusively to professionals" (Havighurst 1990, p. 419). The demand for health care is seen as ineluctably following from the professionally determined "need" for services. Once needs are identified, an appropriate treatment exists. In this spirit the health services research literature speaks of the uninsured as having "unmet needs." Uninsured consumers lack the financial resources to have their needs identified and to obtain treatment for those needs once identified. Health needs—and hence treatment—are determined by medical science; they do not depend on consumer preferences.

This view of health care, which I call a medicalist view, generates a set of allocation and distribution principles entirely different from that of the marketist view. Allocation depends on need, and need is determined by expert providers. In determining need and specifying treatment, individual providers should be guided entirely by medical science and not costs: "Physicians . . . concentrate on medicine" (Himmelstein and Woolhandler 1989, p. 106). In this view acting ethically means disregarding financial rewards and costs (Reinhardt and Relman 1986).

Attaching financial consequences to medical decisions gives providers perverse incentives. The ethical value of disregarding the costs of individual services makes medicalists generally suspicious of most HMOs and other integrated delivery systems that tie physician compensation to the cost of care (Himmelstein and Woolhandler 1989; Mechanic 1992).

To medicalists, government distortions such as the tax subsidy for health insurance are not germane to the problems facing health care. Government programs (whether tax subsidies or direct payments) simply provide consumers with the financial wherewithal to see physicians and have their health needs assessed and met. Ethical providers, freely and independently practicing medicine, will most appropriately allocate health resources. While not all medicalists are physicians (and many physicians are marketists), the medicalist position does depend on a particular view of medical science.

According to the medicalist model, all the information necessary to make decisions is in a patient's diagnosis; prices do not carry valuable information. Instead, prices are simply a vehicle for compensating providers. Medicalists point to the prices that obtain in today's market health system as evidence of the irrelevance of prices as conduits of information. Specialists earn outrageously high salaries, out of proportion to the skill and importance of their efforts. General practitioners, by contrast, earn relatively low and stagnant salaries, although they are on the front lines of medicine, providing preventive and routine care.

The medicalist approach to prices is exemplified by Medicare's Resource-Based Relative Value Scale (RBRVS). Under RBRVS, physicians are paid by Medicare according to a fee schedule based on a scientifically computed point system (De Lew, Greenberg, and Kinchen 1992). The point system measures the skill and effort needed to provide a service. It compensates providers according to the difficulty of the task they undertake, but does not take into account the demand for a provider's product, which, in the medicalist view, is based on the misconceptions of ill-informed consumers. In combination with stringent limitations on billing above the Medicare fee schedule, the implementation of RBRVS means that the prices paid for services rendered by physicians under Medicare have no necessary relationship to those that would emerge from a market equilibrium (Moffit 1992). Instead, the fee schedule compensates providers in proportion to their efforts and rewards evaluation and management functions that the market has disdained.

Prices, in the medicalist view, compensate providers. They can also be manipulated to control the overall costs of the health care system at a "macro" level (Fein 1986). Prices can be used to induce health care spending to conform to levels determined through the political process. Politically determined macro spending limits can be implemented by adjusting fee schedules and deciding what treatments should exist. Decisions to control overall spending are necessary, in the medicalist view, because the high cost of care makes it politically difficult to provide egalitarian coverage for the poor and to meet other social objectives.

Medicalists attribute much of the high cost of care to waste in the system, which they define in terms of unnecessary costs, unnecessary treatments, and, especially, payments to nonproviders—such expenditures as the $18.3 million salary, bonus, and stock option payment made to the chairman of one for-profit hospital chain (Kissick 1994). For medicalists, instances of unnecessary spending include the cost of insurance administration at insurance companies and in doctors' offices, fees paid to lawyers in malpractice cases, and payments to owners of capital, such as the shareholders of insurance companies and for-profit hospitals (Woolhandler and Himmelstein 1991). Marketists celebrate residual claimants (owners of capital) as the engines of producer efficiency, moving their funds to take advantage of new opportunities and providing new and valuable services; medicalists lament the existence of profit in the health care sector. They assert that in a reformed system, "Costs would be constrained by . . . limiting entrepreneurial incentives" (Himmelstein and Woolhandler 1989, p. 106).

The Medicalist Model and the Poor

If, as medicalists argue, health care is unlike other goods, then health care ought to be distributed on a basis different from other goods. While a variety of philosophical principles can justify redistribution of health care—sanctioning the adequacy standard advocated by marketists, for example—the basis of the medicalist approach is egalitarian. The egalitarian argument stems from the position that, "as persons, we are all equally subject to pain, suffering, disability, and death. The need for health care is universal and largely unpredictable" (Dougherty 1988; p. 31). Because need alone determines use, everyone should be entitled to an equitable slice of the health care pie, "where equitable means that the distribution of medical care reflects medical need and the costs and benefits of care" (Fein 1986, p. 194). This position has broad popular appeal. The strictly egalitarian statement that "Everybody should have the right to get the best possible health care—as good as the treatment a millionaire gets" would seem absurd in almost any other context (try substituting food, cars, or housing), but in opinion polls, 90 percent of Americans agreed with it (Jacobs, Shapiro, Schulman 1993, citing a 1990 poll).

This medicalist view is often articulated in terms of a uniform "right" to health care, "the equal access of all citizens to equivalent medical services" (Marmor and Morone 1983, p. 131). American society provides no such egalitarian rights to other goods and services. The quality of food, housing, and higher education purchased by upper-income American families substantially exceeds that bought by the poor. Entitlements to food, housing, and income assistance are restricted to subsets of the population. An egalitarian right to health care can only be justified because health care is different—universally desired and defined by an objective, scientifically determined need, not a subjective preference (Dougherty 1988).

Critiques of the Medicalist Model

The medicalist model's prescription of an egalitarian redistribution of health care has been severely tested by recent developments in health services research. At the foundation of the medicalist model is the assumption that health conditions should determine medically appropriate treatment. But a growing literature examining variations in physician practices suggests that this assumption substantially overstates the connection between condition and treatment.

Variations in practice patterns across the United States and between apparently identical neighboring regions occur for all procedures examined and cannot be explained by simple characteristics of the underlying population or of health resources (Chassin et al. 1987; Leape 1989). Reasonable physicians disagree about appropriate treatment in the vast majority of cases (Eddy and Billings 1988). This interphysician divergence in treatment patterns raises the question of whether an egalitarian "right" to health care should reflect the treatment recommendations of a bold, high-cost physician or those of an equally qualified conservative, low-cost physician.

A growing body of literature also suggests that patients, as well as physicians, differ in their assessment of what constitutes appropriate care in their case (Kasper, Mulley, and Wennberg 1992; Escarce 1993). These studies suggest that given identical symptoms, some patients prefer to live with their condition rather than follow some recommended intervention, once informed of the risks and benefits of treatment. For example, after being given extensive information about treatment, some patients with prostate disease prefer surgery to alleviate their symptoms, while others would bear their symptoms rather than risk the side effects of surgery (Kasper, Mulley, and Wennberg 1992). The importance of patient preferences further weakens the "monotechnic" assumptions of the needs model (Fuchs 1974).

Finally, although much of U.S. health care spending pays for the care of the very ill, most procedures, physician visits, and pharmaceutical treatments address primarily the quality of life, not life expectancy. Even procedures associated with very serious conditions often do more to improve the quality of life than to extend its length. A recent study of heart attack survivors found that those in the United States were twice as likely to receive aggressive treatment (such as bypass surgery) as those in Canada. The two groups had virtually identical 42-month survival rates from the date of the original heart attack. Thirty percent of the Canadian group, however, suffered pain from angina, a rate 25 percent higher than in the United States (Rouleau et al. 1993). The question of whether these Canadian patients "needed" aggressive treatment or not depends on an evaluation of the worth of an enhancement in the quality of life—reduced discomfort from angina. It is not unreasonable to imagine that people vary substantially in their assessment of the value of such a quality-of-life improvement.

The literature also casts doubt on the methods recommended by medicalists for allocating care. Variations in treatment preferences and practices, combined with the continuing development and proliferation of new technologies, make it more difficult to accept the separation of medical decision making from costs that is the policy recommendation of the medicalist model. Where multiple medically acceptable methods of treatment exist and patients have nonmedical reasons for preferring one over another, it is harder to argue that costs should play no part in choosing which to use in a particular case.

Medicalists and the Changing Nature of Medical Care

The existence of multiple rapidly changing modes of treatment casts doubt on the advisability of using administered, rather than market-based, pricing in medical care. Market prices in medical care may not always reflect resource costs very accurately, but the notion "that it is a trivial technical task . . . to set prices in line with costs is belied by the history of administered price systems in all industries, especially those characterized by rapid technological change, as is the case with medical care" (Newhouse 1993b, p. 167).

Organizational innovation exacerbates the problem of administering prices. The very nature of government-administered prices requires that services and facilities be discrete and identifiable. A hospital service is not a physician service. One may be able to come up with different fee schedules for a physician service and a hospital service. In the last ten years, though, medical innovations have made the range of services and facilities multiply. What is a hospital service today? Does it include care in an outpatient facility or a freestanding hospital-related clinic? A service rendered at a freestanding surgery center? Is a hospital different from a "skilled nursing facility"? From an "intermediate care facility"? The regulatory process is necessarily slow, as political and economic factors are weighed in designing regulations. Using administered pricing means freezing into place a particular structure of care provision. It also means endless battles when something that looks like a skilled nursing facility decides it wants to be an intermediate care facility or an outpatient clinic begins providing a service that heretofore had been provided in an inpatient setting.

Recent changes in surgical treatment illustrate this problem. The 1980s saw an explosion of outpatient surgery and freestanding surgical facilities. By 1989 almost half of all surgery took place on an outpatient basis, up from 16 percent in 1980 (CEA 1993). Between 1985 and 1990, the number of freestanding surgical centers certified by Medicare more than doubled to over 1,100 (Sulvetta 1991). Procedures that were once necessarily performed in hospital can now also be performed in a hospital outpatient facility or at a freestanding surgical center. Average costs of procedures performed in these settings differ markedly and unsystematically across procedures and areas (Sulvetta 1991). Furthermore, the relative costs of procedures in each setting are likely to change as resources shift among sites.

The policy recommendation for allocating resources in the medicalist model—economy-wide restrictions on the quantity of health resources combined with government-established provider compensation schedules—is likely to generate substantial allocation mistakes in such a rapidly changing industry. Resources will continue to flow to providers whose services are no longer desired, while new types of providers will find it difficult to establish themselves. This recommendation is inimical to the growth of integrated delivery systems, outpatient surgery, and freestanding surgical facilities, all of which are market responses to changing health care technology.

Given the structure of health spending, marketists are particularly doubtful that the government could successfully make the allocation decisions ceded to it by the medicalist model. The economic theory of regulation suggests that regulation serves the interest of those regulated (Stigler 1971). In a regulated system the biggest spenders and the groups that provide service for them have every incentive to organize and lobby for regulations that protect their interests. Health care policy is shaped by very vocal interest groups—both producers (doctors, hospitals, insurers, drug companies) and certain groups of high-use consumers (the American Association of Retired People [AARP], ACT UP, and so on). The benefits of higher quality and cost health care are very highly concentrated: the top 1 percent of U.S. health care users account for 30 percent of spending in any given year. For this group, health care is their most pressing priority. But the payers for that care include most of the bottom 50 percent of those health spenders who account for just 3 percent of spending (Berk and Monheit 1992). Rising health care costs do cut into their pocketbooks, but for them, health insurance is just one of many concerns. Unlike the organized provider and consumer groups, they have little incentive to lobby Washington for policy changes that reduce costs.

Grafting market mechanisms onto a medicalist structure is just as difficult as combining elaborate redistributive mechanisms with a marketist model. Properly functioning markets require that the possibility of failure exists: producers must suffer the consequences of incorrect decisions, consumers must occasionally be disappointed in their choices (Vladeck 1981). The judicial and political safeguards offered by a government-run system protect participants from failure and undermine market mechanisms (Marmor 1994).

The Debate Today

The debate between medicalists and marketists is not new. Commission reports, books, and scholarly articles throughout this century have argued over the proper allocation and distribution of health care services in similar terms (Starr 1982). In its earlier incarnations the debate drew its fire from the intersection of the venerable dispute over the proper degree of equality in society and a new concern focusing particularly on health care "born of the great strides in medical science made in the late nineteenth century" (Stevens and Stevens 1974, p. 1). As medical training became more standardized, physicians trained in human biology and anatomy agreed on appropriate treatments, and often those treatments worked. With a (relatively) undisputed standard of what medical care was needed in a particular case, the argument for equality received a strong scientific boost (Havighurst 1990).

The latest debate returns to the themes of its predecessors, but with a twist. Where advances in medical science spurred the earlier discussions, an outpouring of research in the social sciences has complicated this one. More is now known about the uncertain meaning of health care "need" and treatment. Experience with public programs has vividly demonstrated the problems of financing care for the poor while medical care changes and costs rise. In place of reasoned arguments, case studies, and survey statistics, this debate is characterized by arcane vocabulary, complex analyses of floods of microdata, grand and costly social experiments, and exhaustive dissections of the programs operating in other nations. The very abundance of information has made action tougher. We know today, much more than before, what does not work. Enough is known about responses to regulations and markets to make policymakers very wary of taking gambles.

Research has undermined both the pure medicalist and pure marketist positions. The disintegration of the poles of the debate should have moved policy attention to the center. Centrists have not made abstract, philosophical arguments. Instead, center ground has been ceded to technocrats who, armed with this accumulation of research, carefully construct elaborate designs intended to address every perverse incentive. Technical solutions, like the Clinton plan, by their nature, are vulnerable to a halfway-effective rhetorical volley from either a marketist or a medicalist.

The special ethical arguments that surround health care policy make any centrist's job even more difficult. Policy advocates have inflamed the health debate with "rights talk." Reformers speak of America's lack of a national health system as a blot on the national character. In the words of one partisan, "what is under discussion is essentially a moral failure, a demonstration of a level of indifference to the well-being of others that stands as an indictment of the intrinsic character of American society" (Rothman 1993, p. 273). Incremental, centrist solutions pale in the face of such zeal.

Opinion poll data show that Americans recognize that health care is mainly a problem for the poor, not for ordinary Americans. A policy solution must address these compassionate, ethical concerns. A successful response to the health sector's ills cannot just solve the problem; it has to talk the talk. But technocratic centrists cannot fall back on principled arguments to explain their amalgam of policy prescriptions. In their concern for dotting every i, they lose sight of any vision to propel their prescriptions forward.

The political system also undermines centrism. Ideological conflicts over the nature of health care compound ordinary lobbying and rivalry over bureaucratic turf, as powerful interest groups and government agencies rally around one or the other viewpoint. The chasm between the two sets of views is so wide, and the opposing views so strongly held, that the two groups find it difficult to enter into thoughtful interchange with each other, let alone agree on a compromise. As one participant in the Clinton task force process put it, arguments over health care often "approach the level of theological disputes" (Kronick 1994, p. 543).

Finally, the conflict between the two positions undermines even incremental reform. All structural reform means making changes to the regulatory infrastructure of health care and almost every such change increases the likelihood that either the marketist or medicalist view of health care will ultimately prevail. Policies that promote competition among managed-care companies alienate supporters of medicalist re-form; policies that enlarge the scope of governmental cost containment enrage marketists. Nobody wants to accept legislation that in any way entrenches the view of the other camp. For each group, doing nothing leaves open the possibility that in the inevitable next round of interest in reform, it will finally be done "right."

3 ///

The Illusion of Inefficiency

If all there was to health reform was raising taxes to pay for care for the uninsured, it seems improbable that so many politicians, including fiscal conservatives, would have championed it. What makes health reform an attractive political issue for both Democrats and Republicans is the idea that it can be accomplished without raising taxes, simply by squeezing waste and inefficiency out of the bloated health care system. Reform, advocates often imply, not only would *not* cost money, but could actually result in net savings. With health reform, middle-class Americans could satisfy their altruistic desire to extend coverage, and reduce the deficit, and spend less on their own health bills.

The size, growth, and nature of the health care sector make the claims of excess credible. Most Americans experience the medical care sector as an occasional visit to a doctor, a visit whose apparent character has hardly changed over time. The static nature of their experience provides little justification for their ever ballooning health insurance premium payments. The few who use specialty services or hospitals may have a greater appreciation of technological change. But they observe an often confusing labyrinth of paperwork, delay, tumult, and uncertainty, equal parts chaos and bureaucracy. Every hospital visitor becomes an instant time-motion expert.

Reform advocates appeal to these popular impressions of squandered dollars and resources, arguing that such waste can be traced to sys-

36

temic—and, more important, correctable—flaws. Medicalists and marketists simply disagree about where the flaws are.

For medicalists, the health sector should be about health care. Waste enters the system through payments to nonproviders or to greedy doctors. These unnecessary expenditures include the costs of insurance administration (among them, payments to insurance companies and to administrators in doctors' offices and hospitals), costs associated with the malpractice system (especially fees paid to lawyers in malpractice cases), skyrocketing compensation for procedure-oriented specialists, and payments to owners of capital, such as the shareholders of insurance companies and for-profit hospitals. As evidence of widespread waste, medicalists point to the significant variations in service utilization across the country and to the growing evidence of inappropriate use of certain procedures. Arguing that these variations demonstrate the need for more scientific rationalization of the health care system, they maintain that better health planning could improve the quality of care while saving money.

For marketists, waste occurs because consumers are insulated from the financial consequences of their service use decisions. Subsidized by government policy, Americans buy overly comprehensive insurance and use services that they do not value at their full cost. The generosity of insurance promotes patterns of care that raise, rather than minimize, cost.

Thousands of anecdotes reinforce the widely held notion of a profligate health sector. It is much harder to trace these excesses to specific and remediable problems. Most of the flaws identified by the medicalists and marketists have little discriminatory power: they point to waste but they do not explain why the health sector should be any more spendthrift than many other parts of the economy. Indeed, many of these apparent problems reflect economy-wide responses to the ever more rapid flow of technology and information, and they therefore surface in other sectors as well. While the methods of managing health care delivery in the United States may differ considerably from those in nations with centrally controlled health care systems, they appear quite similar to those in other sectors of the U.S. economy, sectors that are typically characterized as efficient and vibrant.

Some flaws are particular to health care, but although theoretically plausible, most can account for just a small portion of health costs. The deficiencies fingered by marketists stand up no better to close scrutiny than those fingered by medicalists. Waste, fraud, abuse, and inefficiency undoubtedly exist, but, as I illustrate in this chapter, there is no reason to believe that they are more prevalent in medical care than elsewhere in the economy. Furthermore, there is no reason to believe that any systematic changes in the health sector could significantly reduce these costs over the long run. At best, squeezing inefficiency from the system would yield onetime savings.

Administrative Costs

Most proposals for health reform make at least a gesture in the direction of reducing the administrative costs of the health system. Medicalist reformers, particularly, focus on excessive administrative costs both as a source of potential savings and as a way to undermine the case against an increased government role. If unnecessary paperwork and bureaucracy, customarily perceived as failings of the public sector, are already rampant in the private health care system, perhaps in this sector government intervention could actually reduce bureaucracy as well as costs.

While precise dollar measures of U.S. administrative expenses do not exist, estimates of the full cost of administration (including costs incurred by insurers, in doctors' offices, and in hospitals) suggest that they may comprise as much as 15 percent of total national health spending, $110 billion in 1992 alone (GAO 1992b). The cost of insurance administration—paying bills and managing benefits—comes to about 6 percent of total health spending, up from 4.4 percent of a much smaller total in 1960 (Letsch et al. 1992). Paying bills, collecting revenue from payers, and managing staff are the principal source of provider administrative expenses. Hospitals incurred about $50 billion in administrative costs in 1992, 15 percent of total hospital spending; estimates for physician spending are less precise, but they suggest that more than 10 percent of total physician expenditures may be related to administrative expenses (GAO 1992b). One important component of physician administrative spending is the cost of nonphysician personnel. In 1982 the average doctor's office spent $42,900 on nonphysician personnel. Today the figure is almost 50 percent higher (AMA 1983, 1993).

Administrators make up a large segment of the health sector's labor force. Doctors, nurses, and other professionals who spend time with patients and provide services (such as physical therapists) made up only 28 percent of those employed in the health sector in 1992. About the same number, almost three million people, are employed in administrative-support positions (including managers, accountants, office staff, and lawyers); in 1980 about one million fewer administrative-support staff were employed in health care.[1]

Reformers argue that these rising nonprovider administrative expenditures stem from growing inefficiencies that are specific to the current organization of the health care sector. But while these high and rising levels of administrative employment seem extravagant, they parallel similar patterns in other service industries. Between 1980 and 1992 employment in professional-support occupations in investment banks, law offices, and accounting offices increased by 630,000 people. In percentage terms this increase (77 percent) is larger than the administrative increase in health care (52 percent).[2]

Nor is the level of administrative expenses in health care unusually high. Law firms spent 21 percent of their revenue on nonattorney employee services (including paralegals) in 1992 and an additional 24 percent of their revenue on other overhead costs ("Lawyers' Bottom Line" 1993). In the food industry, administrative expenses (including the costs of marketing and advertising) account for fully 78 percent of total food costs, and they have grown explosively—by 75 percent—since 1981 (Elitzak 1992). Despite this dramatic increase in food administrative expenses, the total cost of food, measured in constant dollars, actually declined about 5 percent over this period (CEA 1993). Throughout the U.S. economy, the percentage of revenue devoted to overhead expenses has risen steadily throughout this century, and especially since 1981. Overhead comprises an average of 20 percent to 35 percent of costs in most industries. In technologically complex sectors, such as pharmaceuticals and electronics, overhead expenses account for almost 75 percent of total costs (Miller and Vollman 1985; Boer 1994). High and rising administrative costs appear to be a feature of the entire U.S. economy, not just the health sector.

Insurance Expenses

The similarity between the pattern of administrative expenses in health care and that in other sectors suggests that the forces leading to rising administrative expenses in health care may not be specific to this particular sector. Nonetheless, it might be desirable to limit administrative costs in health care, even if not in the remainder of the economy, if rising administrative expenses in health care pay for unnecessary services. What do these dollars—and all these people—do?

The most frequently criticized, and most easily measured, portion of administrative costs are the costs incurred by insurance companies. Insurance companies spend money selling policies, pricing policies, paying bills, and managing benefits. While medicalists, who disapprove of private insurance, are the prime critics of insurance expenditures, marketist plans, too, often address insurance costs because these vary tremendously from firm to firm. Marketists see this variation in insurance costs as an opportunity to save money while preserving the structure of private insurance.

Small-group and individual insurance purchasers may pay as much as 40 percent of their insurance premium for administrative costs (CRS 1988). Insurance administration costs for large groups are much lower, averaging 5.5 percent of premiums for the largest firms, only slightly higher than the costs of the federal Medicare program or the Canadian health system. In a small-firm policy, the fixed costs of providing insurance—agent visits, plan design, pricing—must be spread over a small number of covered lives. High failure rates in small firms mean that these costs must also be recouped over a shorter period. Median survival time for small firms that do offer insurance, a more stable subset of all small firms, is only 28 months (Thorpe 1992).

This pattern of costs—higher for small firms than for large firms—also matches that found for other similar purchases. Raw-material costs are often 20 to 25 percent lower in large firms, which can buy in bulk, than in smaller firms. Pension program setup costs are almost twice as high in small firms as in large firms. Consequently, a 10 percent increase in the size of the group covered by a pension plan reduces the per-employee cost of the plan by 6 percent (Brown, Hamilton, and Medoff 1990). Such cost differentials, arising from the higher average cost of selling to smaller units, are not so much a feature of the organization of health care as of the organization of purchasers. Furthermore, the higher costs experienced by smaller firms and individual purchasers have been a feature of the health care market for a long time. In 1959 administrative expenses for individual purchasers comprised as much as 52 percent of total claims costs, while for larger groups the share of administrative expenditures was less than 10 percent (Somers and Somers 1961). It is very unlikely that increases in the cost of selling insurance have contributed substantially to recent increases in health costs.

Money spent assessing someone's health for the purposes of pricing a premium does not pay for any actual health care and may be a source of possible savings. Some argue that the money is not wasted because, by pricing policies, insurers encourage people to engage in healthy behavior. Whatever the case, in aggregate, the dollars do not amount to very much. Very few insurers require people to have a medical examination to obtain coverage; even for individually purchased coverage, fewer than 4 percent of insurers in a recent survey required a special medical examination (OTA 1988). A further 20 percent required that individual purchasers have their physician complete a simple form based on the applicant's medical records. The use of such screening mechanisms declines as the size of the group covered increases. In larger-group contracts, underwriting expenses are very small; after the first year, premium costs can be based on readily available claims experience.

The practice of underwriting small-firm policies has been a source of particular policy concern. Underwriting not only raises costs but may increase premium fluctuations for small businesses (Cutler 1994). When one member of a small group becomes ill, premiums rise for the entire group. These high and volatile costs may discourage small firms from offering insurance to their workers, while raising spending among those who do. In 1991 employees of firms with fewer than 25 workers were only 40 percent as likely to have employer-sponsored health insurance as were employees of firms with 100 or more employees. Sixty-five percent of uninsured workers in 1991 were employed by firms with fewer than 100 employees (Levit, Olin, and Letsch 1992).

The failure of small firms to offer health insurance coverage to their employees, however, does not appear to be closely connected to any special feature of the health insurance market, whether underwriting or high administrative costs. Health insurance may be of special concern to policymakers, but for small firms, it is just another form of employee benefit. As Table 3.1 shows, fewer small firms than large ones provide health coverage to their workers—but small firms are also less likely to offer other fringe benefits, such as life insurance, pensions, paid sick time, and paid vacations.

Insurance marketing expenses, including advertising and agent fees,

Table 3.1   Probability of offering benefits in large firms relative to small firms

Benefit	Ratio of proportion of large firms offering benefit to proportion of small firms offering benefit
Paid vacations	1.63
Health insurance	1.82
Paid sick leave	2.53
Life insurance	3.24
Pensions	4.94

Source: Data from ICF 1987 as reported in Brown, Hamilton, and Medoff 1990.
Note: Large firms have 500 or more employees; small firms have fewer than 500 employees.

are an additional source of administrative costs; they comprise about 9 percent of total administrative expenses (President 1992). Insurers market their products so as to distinguish them from one another. If all insurers produced exactly the same product in exactly the same way, marketing would be completely unnecessary and would not pay. As insurers offer increasingly differentiated products, the cost of conveying their differences to buyers multiply.

To medicalists, who view the differentiation among insurance products as unnecessary, irrelevant, or counterproductive, the costs of advertising these differences are frivolous. Their argument is especially compelling when the main difference among insurers is the healthiness of the populations they cover. But if insurers differentiate themselves by developing distinct ways of cutting costs or monitoring quality, or even by signing up one hospital rather than another in their preferred-provider plan, marketing to convey this information will be as useful in the health insurance industry as in any other industry that develops and improves its products.

The bulk of insurance expenses are for paying bills and, especially, managing benefits (ibid.). This management function has expanded rapidly. In the early 1980s, non-HMO insurers rarely regulated the service utilization of their covered populations (Gray 1991). By 1992, however, the vast majority of non-HMO insurance contracts "managed" benefits in some way (HIAA 1993). In principle, competing insurers will only spend money to manage benefits if they can save more money through reducing the use of services. Existing empirical studies of the effects of preadmission review or utilization review, the most common forms of use management in non-HMO contracts, suggest that many of these programs do save money, net of their administrative costs (Gray 1991; Khandker and Manning 1992). Although providers often complain that utilization review organizations save this money by indiscriminately limiting use, a study of the industry suggests that such review programs typically employ skilled reviewers (registered nurses) and use physicians and specialists to evaluate claims that are appealed (GAO 1993a). Furthermore, since 1990 utilization review organizations have been accredited by independent organizations that in effect monitor the monitors (ibid.; Smith 1993). To the extent that utilization review reduces the provision of unnecessary services, the administrative costs associated with these programs may both save money and lead to higher quality.

The significant and growing role of utilization management in administration costs exemplifies the pitfalls of assessing the efficiency of the health care system through the share spent on administration. Higher administrative costs do not necessarily mean higher health costs. Cross-country comparisons support this view. As Figure 3.1 shows, in data from the Organization for Economic Cooperation and Develop-

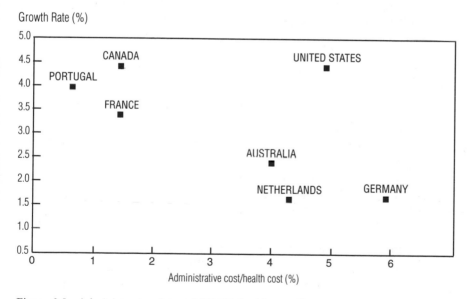

Figure 3.1   Administrative share of OECD health spending, 1980, and growth of OECD health spending, 1980–1990. Growth rates shown are the real per capita rates for each nation adjusted by its GDP deflator. (*Source:* OECD 1993b.)

ment (OECD) there appears to be a negative correlation between administrative expenses per capita and the rate of growth in health spending per capita in developed countries. Germany, which has the highest costs of insurance administration among all OECD countries reporting expenses, has also been more successful than any other major industrialized country in reducing overall growth in health care cost during the 1980s.

As treatment choices in health care multiply, most health care systems outside the United States have reformed their systems to add administrative costs in the form of tighter control of utilization. Germany has more rigorous utilization review (GAO 1993a), some Canadian provinces now monitor individual physician receipts quarterly (OECD 1993a), and the British system now gives doctors responsibility for their referrals ("Survey of Healthcare" 1991). In each case policymakers expect the savings from reduced utilization to outweigh any increase in administrative costs.

Provider Administrative Costs

Reformers argue that the costs of insurance administration, the only administrative costs enumerated in the national health accounts, grossly understate the administrative burden generated by the U.S. multipayer health system. Most health administrators work for providers, not insurance companies. The element of provider costs most affected by the U.S. multipayer system is the cost of billing payers. Like other firms, providers must cope with cash, check, and credit card payments, although most health bills are paid by a limited number of insurers, rather than a large number of distinct clients as in other industries. Physician billing costs also increase with the number of different payers in each physician's practice and with the number of patients who are required to pay a share of their own bills. Conservative estimates of billing-related provider costs suggest that they may have amounted to as much as $36 billion in 1991 (President 1992).

Even this conservative figure may overstate the importance of billing costs. If these costs were an important contributor to overall costs, one would expect to see that differences in organizational structure that raise or lower billing costs would be associated with differences in the level of costs and the rate of cost growth. The growing market share of insurers that contract with providers (such as preferred-provider organizations and health maintenance organizations) during the 1980s should have reduced billing costs. Billing costs of providers who contracted with a small number of insurers should have decreased relative to those of noncontracting providers, who continued to face many different payers.

Instead, overall expenditures for support personnel rose during the 1980s and the pattern within sectors was similar. The nonphysician expenses of physicians in solo practice, who are less likely to contract with managed-care companies than group practice physicians, should have been expected to grow relative to those of group practice physicians (Dynan 1994). But the nonphysician personnel costs of group practice physicians actually grew faster than those of solo practitioners during the 1980s (AMA 1983, 1993).

States with regulated, centralized payment systems have lower billing costs than less regulated states. Hospital billing costs in New York, where a single billing form is used and all private payers pay regulated rates, are among the lowest in the United States, and only slightly higher than billing costs in Canada (PROPAC 1993). Billing costs in California may be as high as 20 percent of total costs (Thorpe 1992). Yet hospital costs per capita in New York are much higher than those in California and grew much faster than costs in California during the 1980s (Zwanziger et al. 1993).

Overhead costs have grown throughout the hospital sector, both in states with diverse payment arrangements and in those with simple ones. Between 1980 and 1992, nonphysician employment in hospitals grew as quickly (per inpatient day) in Maryland and New York, where all private payers pay the same rates and use the same billing forms, as in California and Minnesota, where hospitals bid for contracts from multiple insurers, and as in the United States as a whole, where a diversity of payment arrangements exists (see Table 3.2). If these additional personnel were mainly needed to perform labor-intensive billing tasks, the share of labor in total hospital expenses would also have grown. Instead, the share of labor in total hospital expenses declined in all four states and in the country as a whole.

The effects on total costs of differences in overhead expenses do not support the hypothesis that rising overhead costs explain much of rising health spending. Furthermore, the composition of nonphysician em-

Table 3.2 Changes in hospital administrative costs by state, 1980–1992

Jurisdiction	Labor costs as a share of total costs			Nonphysician personnel per 100 bed days		
	1980 share	1992 share	Change in share	1980 count	1992 count	Change in count
California	57.0	53.9	−5.44%	1.07	1.52	42.1%
Minnesota	60.9	57.6	−5.42	0.80	1.10	37.5
New York	63.7	61.2	−3.92	0.78	1.14	46.2
Maryland	61.1	57.5	−5.89	0.85	1.43	68.2
United States	59.0	54.9	−6.95	0.89	1.41	58.4

Source: American Hospital Association, 1981, 1993.
Note: Figures are based on full-time salaried employees (including RNs and LPNs).

ployment in health care has also changed in a direction that suggests that rising billing costs cannot explain much of the increase in health costs. During the 1980s hospitals decreased the share of their employees who were less skilled and increased their employment of highly skilled registered nurses and physical therapists (PROPAC 1993). International evidence buttresses the view that changes in hospital care, not administrative expenses, led to this shift. The number of staff per hospital bed increased between the early and late 1980s in 15 of the 16 countries (other than the United States) for which the OECD has collected data.[3]

The rising skill level of administrative employment and the parallel growth in nonphysician employment under a variety of organizational structures suggest that changes in the function of administrators and nonphysician staff, rather than the nature of the U.S. multipayer system itself, explain rising administrative and nonphysician expenses. One such new function is the provider portion of utilization review. Hospital and physician billing departments increasingly have to justify the services that they have provided or plan to provide. Justifying bills, in turn, means keeping more complete documentation of both services and the symptoms and diagnoses that prompted them. Without further training, billing clerks are unlikely to be able to perform these functions.

But providers also need more administrators and other staff to cope with the rising flood of information that passes through their offices. If patients undergo more tests, or have them performed sooner, administrators must process more paper, faster. If referrals encompass a larger array of subspecialists, or a larger selection of physicians who participate in a variety of insurance arrangements, more cross-references must be kept. If patients can be treated in more diverse settings, price and quality records about these venues must be maintained. If new technologies, treatments, or guidelines are developed at an accelerated pace, someone must keep track of the changes.

Such rapid technological change in other sectors has also been associated with increases in skill levels and with an increase in the proportion of employment that is supervisory, administrative, or managerial rather than service- or goods-producing (Miller and Vollman 1985; Bartel and Lichtenberg 1987). The administrative costs of health care are likely to continue increasing as long as the institutional structure of the health system accommodates technological change.

The evidence suggests that rising administrative costs do not stem from flaws peculiar to the health sector and do not make an important contribution to total health care costs. Estimates for 1991 of the potential aggregate effect on health care costs of moving to a system with minimal administrative costs, such as a single-payer system, range from a savings of $69 billion (assuming that there is no additional utilization from the elimination of all patient copayments and utilization review among the currently insured) to an additional cost of $60 billion (assuming that these utilization control measures have a substantial effect on use; GAO 1992b). These estimates were computed under the assumption that coverage would be extended to the uninsured (although they do not include the costs of such coverage). If coverage were not extended, administrative savings would be smaller than these figures indicate, since providers would continue to incur the billing costs associated with self-paying patients.

None of these estimates incorporates potential effects of reductions in administrative costs on the growth and transformation of the health sector. The similarities between the growth of administrative costs in health care and in other sectors suggest that higher administrative costs may be a sensible response to rapidly changing technologies and organizational forms: a consequence of limiting the use of questionable procedures, helping providers select less costly forms of care, and informing consumers of their health care options. If so, reducing administrative expenses today could raise the aggregate cost of a given quality of care as health provision changes in the future. Potential administrative savings at a point in time pale when compared to changes over time in health care costs. Even the highest estimate of potential administrative savings is only about 70 percent as large as the real difference in national health spending between 1990 and 1991.[4]

Malpractice

Most Americans believe that malpractice awards are too high. In polls 59 percent say that the malpractice system contributes "a great deal" to the nation's health care problems (Sage, Hastings, and Berenson 1994). Responding to these perceptions, most states have undertaken reforms of their malpractice litigation systems, and malpractice modifications figure in most federal reform proposals (OTA 1993a). In 1991 malpractice insurance premiums, which reflect the cost of actual awards and settlements and most of the cost of litigation, amounted to $9 billion (AHA 1992). Litigation costs—fees paid to lawyers—alone account for about 40 percent of the total costs of malpractice (CEA 1993).

These costs, while high, account for less than 1 percent of national health expenditures directly (OTA 1993a). But the malpractice system increases costs indirectly by encouraging the spread of "defensive medicine"—practices designed to minimize the risk of a successful lawsuit. Studies sponsored by the American Medical Association suggest that about $20 billion was spent on defensive medical practices in 1989, almost 20 percent of physician expenditures, and 4 percent of total health costs (Moser and Musacchio 1991). Malpractice insurance costs have also been growing at astronomical rates. Between 1982 and 1989, malpractice premiums increased 15 percent annually, much more rapidly than total health expenditures (CEA 1993).

These substantial costs, however, pale against the enormous cost of injuries caused by malpractice. Despite the size of the malpractice industry, most people who are negligently injured through medical practice are never compensated. Two studies, one conducted in California in 1974 and one conducted in New York in 1984, looked at hospital records to identify injuries that might have been caused by negligence and tracked the disposition of these cases (Danzon 1985; Weiler et al.

1993). In the California study, 1 in 126 hospital admissions suffered an injury attributable to negligence. One in 10 of those injured actually made a claim for compensation. In the New York study, 1 in 8 of those negligently injured claimed compensation. In the California study, only 1 in 25 of those injured negligently actually obtained compensation. In New York, 1 in 15 received compensation.

Total payments to injured plaintiffs amount to about $4 billion annually, roughly 40 to 45 percent of the $9 billion in U.S. malpractice premiums collected each year (Weiler 1991; AHA 1992). Even if one assumes that those who sued had injuries four times as serious as those who did not sue, the figures from California and New York suggest that the cost that would have been incurred nationally to compensate all those injured through malpractice in 1991 was about $20 billion.[5] Although there are serious deficiencies in the malpractice system, any alternative system that sought proper compensation for most of those injured through medical negligence would be at least as costly (White 1994).

The failure of the malpractice system to compensate those injured is echoed by its failure to deter further negligence. A very tiny fraction of doctors account for a substantial fraction of suits and an even larger fraction of suits won by plaintiffs. In 1987 and 1988, 6 percent of anesthesiologists and obstetricians in one sample were responsible for 85 percent of all malpractice awards in these specialty groups (Sloan et al. 1989). Furthermore, the same physicians are sued over and over again. Within specialty, physicians in one study who had lost a malpractice case were almost three times more likely than other physicians to have been sued again (Bovbjerg and Petronis 1994).

Although malpractice awards are highly concentrated, the structure of the malpractice insurance system assures these physicians that their premiums will not rise disproportionately. Unlike auto insurance, where an individual's premiums rise significantly when that person's claims increase, malpractice insurance as a rule is very weakly experience-rated within each specialty group (Sloan 1990). The community-rated nature of malpractice insurance means that when one physician persistently behaves negligently, all physicians in that group see an increase in their premiums. Empirical studies show that most of the increase in the cost of malpractice insurance premiums is then passed along to patients (Danzon, Pauly, and Kington 1990). Rising malpractice costs do not affect physician incomes or discourage negligent physicians from practicing.

While malpractice litigation may not deter bad doctors from practicing, it could actually improve the quality of care (while raising costs) by encouraging the practice of appropriate, negligence-reducing "defensive medicine." According to the AMA study, most physicians report making extra notations in charts, ordering additional diagnostic tests, referring complex cases to specialists, and talking to patients more as their most frequent defensive-medicine activities (Reynolds, Rizzo, and Gonzalez 1987). Although these activities may raise the costs of medical practice, they seem to be precisely the kinds of behaviors that would reduce the incidence of costly negligent behavior.

Even the most liberal estimates of the costs of defensive medicine and malpractice insurance find that they cannot account for more than 6 percent of U.S. health care costs (premiums plus 20 percent of physician practice costs), less than one year's worth of growth in inflation-adjusted cost (Moser and Musacchio 1991). Nor can they explain any significant portion of rising health care costs. In fact, in the late 1980s, malpractice premiums actually began to decline, falling almost 30 percent in constant dollars between 1988 and 1992 (OTA 1993a). A complete evaluation of the U.S. malpractice system should not rest on the effect of the system on direct medical costs, however, but on its effectiveness in deterring poor physicians and compensating those who are injured. On these criteria the system fails dismally. Despite the fuss over large awards and costly defensive practices, poor physicians are not forced out of the market by malpractice and most injured patients are not compensated.

Many states have passed legislation aimed at reducing malpractice costs, mainly by capping awards (OTA 1993a). Unfortunately, these reforms of the malpractice system seem unlikely to reduce *total* health costs—that is, those that include the actual costs of injuries to plaintiffs. Legislation limiting malpractice awards for pain and suffering appears to have had some effect on the size of malpractice awards, but this approach does not improve the system's success at either compensating the negligently injured or deterring negligent practice.

Some scholars have argued that medical associations and licensing boards should do a better job of regulating the profession (Fuchs 1994c). These boards already have the power to discipline persistently negligent physicians and prevent them from practicing. In the past, though, medical associations have been extremely reluctant to police their own. In 1989 fewer than 3,000 of the more than 600,000 physicians practicing in the United States were disciplined in any way, and only half this number had their licenses suspended or revoked or were put on probation (VanTuinen, McCarthy, and Wolfe 1991).[6] By contrast, malpractice insurers sanctioned more than 1.25 percent of those they insured. Complaint procedures discourage patients from raising concerns. Even where egregious misconduct is discovered, penalties are often minimal. Many medical boards do not even specify incompetence as grounds for delicensure (Gaumer 1984).

Better discipline by medical societies might reduce negligent behavior, but it would not compensate those who are injured nonetheless. Reforms of the tort system that provide more efficient ways of compensating plaintiffs injured through negligence might also be desirable, but in the absence of significant reform of the self-policing system, such reforms might eliminate even the limited deterrence capacity that malpractice law now provides (White 1994). Without better monitoring and incentives that encourage physicians to take appropriate defensive precautions, medical malpractice reform could increase national health-related costs, not reduce them.

The increasing corporatization of medical practice may provide one way to improve the functioning of the malpractice system, at least with respect to deterrence. If insurers are sued for the damages caused by the physicians on their preferred-provider lists, they will be particularly careful in selecting and monitoring the quality of care provided by these physicians. Increasing the liability of insurers for the care they pay for would also serve as a useful counterbalance to insurer interests in reducing the cost of care.

The Clinton health task force working group on malpractice reform proposed a reform called "enterprise liability" as a way of encouraging such a development. An enterprise liability system would move responsibility for physician misconduct to the level of the insurer or HMO that paid for the care (Sage, Hastings, and Berenson 1994). Enterprise liability would encourage insurers and HMOs to employ more careful monitoring of the quality of services provided by the physicians they reimbursed. Many physician groups, insurers, and lawyers were appalled by the notion of enterprise liability. Physicians rightly saw it as added incentive for insurers to encroach on doctors' traditional autonomy. Insurers recognized that they did not have the capacity to monitor the behavior of physicians. Lawyers sensed that demand for their services might shrink in a more concentrated system. Finally, states were concerned that this new rule encroached on their constitutional role of managing intrastate civil litigation.

The Clinton administration's final proposals on malpractice reform were much more circumscribed. Enterprise liability would have gone forward only as a demonstration project. Lawyers' contingency fee rates would be limited, standards of proof for filing a suit would be strengthened, and mechanisms for the resolution of disputes outside the courts would be enhanced. These proposals are a minimalist version of most standard malpractice-reform proposals, which focus on limiting the magnitude of awards and the scope of claims. The Bush administration proposal, for example, would have capped noneconomic damages and eliminated joint and several liability for noneconomic damages. Although this kind of reform is popular among physician groups, it does little to ensure that more of those injured are compensated or to deter physicians from practicing negligently.

The Insurance Industry

Medicalists dislike the multipayer insurance system in part because it generates administrative expenses. They find even more disturbing, though, the idea that the private insurance system, like other for-profit institutions within health care, operates for the benefit of its shareholders. Medicalists are particularly troubled that insurers generate these profits in part by denying coverage to those in ill health. Even if the expenses incurred by private insurers work to keep other costs down or to encourage innovation in health services, the profits generated by insurers seem less justifiable as a source of health insurance premium costs.

Today, there are about 1,000 private insurers offering health insurance coverage in the United States (De Lew, Greenberg, and Kinchen 1992). In total, health insurers collected $255.5 billion in premiums for health insurance in 1991 (HIAA 1993). While profits fluctuate from year to year, an estimate for 1991, a relatively profitable year, suggests that they comprise no more than 5 percent of insurer administrative costs and less than 0.3 percent of national health expenditures (President 1992).

Even these figures overstate the role of profits in raising health sector costs. Reported profitability data suggest that the industry's fortunes follow a cycle of about three years as firms enter the industry in profitable years and close down when they incur losses. Underwriting profits in many years are lower than those in 1991, and periods of losses have typically followed periods of profit (Gabel et al. 1991, 1994). The ease of entry and exit into this industry suggests that sustained profits are unlikely.

Most of those "profits" do not accrue to traditional investors. Very little of the insurance sold in the United States is sold by stockholder-capitalized insurance companies. Although their market share has been shrinking, the Blue Cross/Blue Shield companies, private, not-for-profit insurers, still sell about 40 percent of all the private insurance contracts in the United States (HIAA 1993). The three largest HMOs, too, are not-for-profit (GHAA 1994). More than 30 percent of Americans obtain insurance through their self-insured employers and have no connection to the commercial insurance market (HIAA 1993). Among the commercial health insurers who cover the remainder, about 40 percent are mutual insurance companies (GAO 1986). The largest seller of individual policies, Mutual of Omaha, and the largest seller of group insurance plans, Prudential, are both mutual companies (*Best's* 1992). In a mutual insurance company, the shareholders are the policyholders themselves. Any profits that accrue to the company are turned back to policyholders in the form of lower premiums or dividends. Only a small minority of Americans buy insurance premiums from stock companies that earn profits for autonomous shareholders.

Overall, these data suggest that insurance industry profits are unlikely either to drive health costs or add substantially to the level of costs. But this evidence alone does not address the question of why any profits should be permitted in this industry. While profits may not be important today, for-profit companies are capturing an increasing share of the health care market, especially in managed care (GHAA 1994). Do these profits serve a useful purpose?

Business profits represent a return on capital invested in an industry.[7] Without offering such a return, insurers would be forced to finance their operations through debt (which pays interest to bondholders and savers) or forgo investing altogether. The role of profits in attracting new capital means that publicly traded for-profit insurers are likely to expand still further as the management of care becomes a more important part of the industry. Insurers need new funds to establish the infrastructure to review claims, develop guidelines for claims payment, and process information (Galt 1994). For-profit insurers, who can turn to the equity market for these funds, will find it easiest to enter new markets. A well-functioning capital market, in turn, should reward innovative insurers who develop new and better products.

Innovation in the health insurance industry had, until recently, been rather circumscribed. In the past ten years, insurers have made significant and novel changes in their relationships with their providers. As yet, the relationship between insurers and customers and the position of health insurers in the capital markets has changed much less. State insurance regulators, who monitor the finances of insurance companies, and financial-market regulations that limit the insurance activities of other financial intermediaries, may have slowed the rate of innovation in this sector (Cochrane 1995).

The effect of heavy regulation on the insurance side of the industry has encouraged insurers to skew their innovation efforts toward managing care—an arena that, until now, has almost completely escaped regulation. There has been far less innovation in the design of new insurance products with features that would appeal to individual purchasers, small groups, or the self-employed.[8] In part, delays in developing such products may have occurred because insurance regulators, responsible for ensuring that insurers do not become insolvent and call on state insurance guaranty funds, have required firms to charge premiums high enough to cover expected payouts and to maintain reserve funds large enough for most contingencies. These regulations may make it quite difficult, for example, to offer a multiyear insurance contract. Such regulations have protected consumers from insolvent insurers, but they may also have retarded the development of new and desirable insurance products (McDowell 1989; Galt 1994).

The slow rate of financial innovation in the insurance market resembles the situation of the financial-services sector before deregulation of that industry in the mid-1970s. Since deregulation, the financial-services sector has developed hundreds of new products, which permit the diversification and better allocation of many risks. Today, investment banking firms attract "some of the brightest talent the United States has to offer . . . and reward the producers and players handsomely. The industry attracts creative people, self-starters, entrepreneurs, and risk takers" (Galt 1994, p. 275). By contrast, highly regulated financial-services sectors, such as insurance, tend to employ more conservative and bureaucratic employees.

These revolutionary changes have meant significant losses for some investors, but they have also led to a tremendous increase in the ability of the U.S. financial sector to identify and provide capital for new investment. The financial-services sector has even begun to innovate within health insurance. Today, health insurance futures and options are traded on the Chicago Stock Exchange (Hayes, Cole, and Meisleman 1993; Russ 1993). In principle these trades allow insurance companies and firms to protect themselves against the risk of unexpectedly high health insurance costs. Deregulation and increased competition in health insurance could unleash a flood of new, and potentially better, insurance products—although, as in financial services, deregulation would undoubtedly bring new, and significant, dangers of insurer failure.

For-Profit Providers

The increasing role of for-profit entities in providing health care, not just health insurance, is troubling to many medicalists. As one critic put it, "It does take the breath away—at least it takes away mine—to see clearly that in the present state of affairs, the profits gained from the practice of medicine appear to show up in the pockets of speculators" (Wohl 1984, p. 17).

For-profit behavior in medicine is nothing new. Most independent physicians provide care "for profit," keeping the excess of revenues over costs as their earnings from practice. Medicalists argue that independently practicing physicians balance their professional ethics against their pocketbook interests.[9] But the growing role of third-party shareholders in the industry raises concerns that decisions made to enrich shareholders could hurt patients. These concerns are long-standing. The Committee on the Costs of Medical Care, writing in 1932, inveighed against for-profit providers, arguing that "lay groups organized for profit have no legitimate place" providing medical services (Committee 1932, p. 48).

The advantages and disadvantages of for-profit providers can be seen most clearly in the case of the hospital industry, where a majority of providers are not-for-profit. Not-for-profit hospitals, which do not pay dividends to shareholders, are exempt from most taxes in return for providing services, often ill defined, to their local communities. While the managers of for-profit hospitals must ultimately answer to their shareholders, the chain of command in not-for-profits is murkier. In some cases, sponsoring institutions, such as religious or charitable groups, may exert strong control over the hospital; in others, hospitals are run primarily by their senior staff physicians.

Studies of the relative costs of for-profit and not-for-profit hospitals typically find little difference between them (Gray 1991). Profits paid to shareholders do not appear to increase the cost of for-profit hospitals significantly. At the same time, there is little evidence that not-for-profits manage their operations wastefully (Becker and Sloan 1985). Like other managers, not-for-profit hospital managers try to operate their hospitals efficiently, by keeping costs down and revenues high. But instead of distributing the excess of revenues over costs to shareholders, they disperse it in other ways, either by providing care to indigent patients (as they are obliged to do in some states) or by providing other community services. On average, about 6 percent of the care provided by not-for-profit hospitals is uncompensated (House Ways and Means Committee 1992).

The government's financial support of non-profits (through the tax system) serves as a way of compensating them for this traditional role of providing care for the indigent. This rationale, though, has less salience in a world accustomed to Medicaid, Medicare, and formal uncompensated care payment mechanisms than it did in the nineteenth century. Recognizing this change, an Internal Revenue Service ruling in 1969 removed the requirement that not-for-profit hospitals provide charity care in order to retain their tax-exempt status (Burns 1973). Furthermore, the burden of uncompensated care is spread very unevenly among not-for-profit hospitals. In some not-for-profit hospitals, most patients are indigent; in others, virtually no patients are unable to pay their bills (Lewin, Eckels, and Miller 1988). Most studies find that for-profit hospitals see fewer uncompensated patients than not-for-profits, but among nonteaching hospitals the difference is primarily due to differences in the locations of for-profit and not-for-profit hospitals rather than in their treatment of individual patients (Gray 1991; Norton and Staiger 1994). Public hospitals bear most of the burden of caring for the uninsured (Coffey 1983).

In theory, not-for-profits, who seek to satisfy doctors and local communities rather than shareholders, may put the extra earnings they do not spend on indigent care into higher-quality services (Pauly 1987). Limited empirical evidence from the nursing-home market suggests that for-profit organizations in that sector may provide lower-quality care than not-for-profit organizations (Gertler 1989).[10] The theoretical and empirical evidence suggests that not-for-profits are no more prone to waste money than are for-profits. In a snapshot view, a shift toward a more profit-oriented industry seems, on balance, like a mistake.

But the picture becomes more cloudy when examined over time. The hospital industry is at the tail end of a wrenching transition. The use of inpatient hospital care plummeted in the 1980s. Admissions per capita fell 25 percent and the average length of stay per admission fell by 0.8 days, from 7.1 to 6.3 days. The combination of reduced admissions and shorter stays drove bed days in U.S. hospitals down almost 40 percent between 1980 and 1990. The effect on capacity utilization in the industry was dramatic. On the average day in 1980, 75.5 percent of U.S. short-stay hospital beds were occupied. Almost 500 short-stay hospitals in the U.S. closed during the 1980s. Nonetheless, by the early 1990s, occupancy rates hovered between 60 and 65 percent in the remaining 5,400 hospitals (DHHS, various years).

These declines were the result of changes both in payment patterns and technologies. The main change in payments was the implementation of a prospective payment method in the Medicare system. In 1983 Medicare, the largest single payer to U.S. hospitals, switched from paying on a per diem basis to making a lump sum payment according to a patient's principal diagnosis, or DRG. This prospective payment system provides incentives for hospitals to treat patients as economically as possible (which often means discharging them sooner) and makes it harder for hospitals to recoup expenses by charging separately for each service rendered.

The introduction of prospective payment coincided with the development of a number of new technologies for outpatient surgery and diagnosis. In 1980 two of the four most frequently performed procedures for men over sixty-five in U.S. hospitals were repair of inguinal hernia and extraction of lens (cataract surgery). By 1990 the rates of inpatient inguinal hernia operations in this group had dropped by half and inpatient cataract surgery had declined by almost 90 percent (DHHS, various years). The preponderance of these procedures are now performed on an outpatient basis.

The proliferation of outpatient surgical techniques transformed the hospital from a place where many people went for short episodes of treatment to a site where only more serious cases were treated. The staple treatments of the 1970s moved to new facilities. Many procedures moved to outpatient departments of existing hospitals, where payment methods are less stringent. Others moved out of hospitals altogether.

In another industry, such low-capacity usage, with no reasonable expectations of a significant increase in demand soon, would lead to massive declines in capacity. In the steel industry, for example, a 45 percent decline in production between 1978 and 1982, about twice as large as the decline in hospital days between 1980 and 1985, led to the retirement of over 25 percent of steel-producing capacity between 1982 and 1988 (GAO 1989b). By contrast, only 6 percent of U.S. hospital beds were taken out of service between 1985 (the peak of occupancy) and 1991.

Most not-for-profit hospitals have their roots in local charitable or religious organizations or in the local physician population. They view themselves, and are viewed, as community institutions. Hospital employees and local politicians alike gain from maintaining existing hospitals. A hospital is often the largest employer in a small town, as well as an important selling point in attracting new businesses and residents. Closing hospitals is often politically infeasible. Their sense of place means that they do not close up and move as their communities do, a problem identified by the mid-1930s (Stevens 1989).

The converse is also true. New suburbs and communities gain non-profit beds only slowly, as community organizations arise and gain the resources to support them. Unlike a corporation that relocates its headquarters, a declining not-for-profit hospital cannot simply move to a new site and provide service to a new community. For-profit institutions can more readily match the growth of new communities. Ironically, in the 1930s, the same combination of forces meant that for-profit hospitals were more likely than not-for-profits to be located in poorer communities. These communities contained enough paying patients to cover the cost of medical services and keep a hospital operating, but they could not amass the charitable resources to fund the establishment of a new hospital (Stevens 1989).

For-profit institutions, precisely because they respond to impersonal capital markets rather than local community pressure, may adapt better than not-for-profits do to rapid changes in technology, payments, preferences, and institutions. In 1986, when occupancy rates in hospitals dropped precipitously, shareholders responded by squeezing 20 percent of the funds out of the for-profit hospital industry, in effect forcing changes in hospital behavior (Smith 1986). Between 1985 and 1987, for-profit hospitals increased the share of surgery performed on an outpatient basis by almost 40 percent, somewhat more than either private not-for-profit or state and locally run hospitals (my calculations, based on data in DHHS 1993).

The development of outpatient techniques, which devastated the in-patient hospital industry, created new opportunities for for-profit enterprises and spawned a new institution, the freestanding surgical and diagnostic center. By 1990 at least 1,696 of such centers existed in the United States (Smith 1993). The first outpatient surgical clinic was opened by an entrepreneurial surgeon in the mid-1970s (Ginzberg and Ostow 1994). Today, almost all freestanding clinics operate for profit.

Deciding whether a shift toward a more profit-oriented health system is good or bad depends on one's characterization of the system. Not-for-profits provide more service to the indigent and more responsiveness to local community pressures; some literature in the nursing-home sector suggests that they may provide higher-quality services, albeit at higher cost. For-profits are quicker to respond to population movements and to the development of technologies that require new institutions or organizational structures. The virtues of not-for-profits will diminish if more people have their care paid for by insurance, rather than relying on free care, and as more attention is paid to the objective measurement of hospital quality. It seems likely that nonprofessional shareholders will play an increasing part in the U.S. health system, but there is no evidence that such a change would raise the costs of the system or substantially change the nature and quality of care provided.

Doctors

Multiple competing insurers, the malpractice system, and proprietary medical institutions are the front line of the medicalists' critique of the current U.S. health care sector. But medicalists also see room for improvement—and savings—within the traditional health sector, particularly in the compensation of physicians.

Payments directly to physicians account for 19 percent of U.S. health spending. Between 1980 and 1990 these payments increased by $65 billion, to $134 billion—an astonishing 94 percent rise. Payments to physicians accounted for 20 percent of the increase in national health spending in the 1980s (Letsch et al. 1992).

Part of the increase in spending paid for the rising cost of physician practice. Average expenses for physicians, including rapidly escalating malpractice premium costs, rose by 50 percent in real terms over the decade (Pope and Schneider 1992). Physicians, like hospitals, invested heavily in medical technology over the decade.

The increases in practice expenses explain only a portion of the rise in physician payments. Over the period from 1982 through 1992, real incomes of physicians, net of practice expenses, rose 25 percent (AMA 1993). While income growth has slowed substantially since 1989, physicians began the decade of the 1980s as the highest-paid occupational group in America—earning about 4.5 times as much as the average worker—and ended it in an even stronger position: by 1990, the average physician earned more than 5 times as much as the average American (CBO 1993c). The 600,000 practicing American physicians earned an average of $172,000 (before taxes) in 1992 (AMA 1993). They are the most highly paid physicians in the world, both in absolute terms (they earn about 70 percent more than Canadian physicians, who are the next-best paid) and in relative terms (CBO 1993c).[11]

Marketists argue that the reason physicians earn so much is that the government has made entry into the physician market very difficult. Physicians, as a group, have some characteristics of a cartel. A potent political force in America, organized medicine has blocked reform efforts that would reduce doctors' earnings and has controlled entry into the profession (Starr 1982; Friedman and Kuznets 1945). Practicing physicians license newly trained doctors in each state and may choose to restrict entry (through higher test score requirements, longer educational periods, or limits on places in medical schools) in order to maintain the quality of practice or to strengthen the cartel (Sarkar 1995). Recent declines in physician compensation have led to further attempts to solidify the cartel, this time by blocking the entry of foreign-trained medical graduates (Institute of Medicine 1995). In the past, state physician associations have also succeeded in disciplining physicians who attempted to compete by offering prepaid services (Starr 1982).

The cartel power of physicians suggests that at a point in time, the price of physician services is likely to be higher than would exist in a purely competitive market. That is, physicians are likely to be earning economic rents—returns higher than they could achieve in an alternative occupation. In addition to their power to control entry, physicians can, to some degree, influence the extent of demand for their services. Physicians can recommend diagnostic tests, follow-up visits, or other services of equivocal necessity to raise their incomes. This pattern is common to many service industries in which customers are not fully informed about the costs and benefits of treatment: car mechanics recommend additional, possibly unnecessary, servicing, hairdressers recommend hot-oil treatments, investment brokers churn accounts. In the health services literature, the practice is known as physician-induced demand.[12]

But cartel power and demand inducement cannot explain the rapid increase in physician incomes in the 1980s. The decline in traditional fee-for-service insurance and the growth of managed care and PPO-type arrangements, combined with a decline in membership in the physicians' main professional organization, the American Medical Association, has meant that the power of the physician cartel has weakened (Noether 1986). As physicians have competed with one another for coveted positions on preferred-provider lists, the cartel's power to maintain prices has eroded.[13] Demand inducement has been limited by the growth of utilization review and capitation payment. All in all, the rise of managed care in the 1980s ought to have led to a reduction in cartel power and demand inducement—and hence physician incomes— not an increase.

The cartel and induced-demand explanations rely on peculiar characteristics of the physician market that do not seem to have been operating strongly in the 1980s. But the growth in earnings experienced by physicians in the decade paralleled similar growth in earnings for other highly skilled professionals. The incomes of other professional groups rose about as much during the 1980s as did average incomes of physicians: accountants' incomes rose 19 percent, lawyers' incomes rose 27 percent, college professors' incomes rose 30 percent (Pope and Schneider 1992).[14]

The most plausible explanation for higher physician earnings is simply an increase in the demand for the services of these highly skilled workers without a corresponding increase in supply. Almost all of the increase in average physician incomes during the 1980s occurred among the most highly trained physicians, medical specialists; between 1983 and 1988, average incomes for surgeons grew 39 percent and medical specialists' incomes rose 30 percent. General practitioners' incomes, expressed in real terms, rose only 14 percent in this period (Pope and Schneider 1992). Economists have described similar patterns of earnings growth during the 1980s among the most skilled within occupations throughout the American economy (Juhn, Murphy, and Pierce 1993).

The growth in earnings was concentrated in a limited number of specialties where new techniques had been recently developed and the number of practicing specialists had not grown as much. The greatest income growth between 1983 and 1988 occurred among cardiologists (53 percent), orthopedic surgeons (63 percent), ophthalmologists (43 percent), and cardiovascular surgeons (measured imprecisely at over 100 percent). The 1980s saw explosive growth in the use of coronary artery bypass surgery (performed by cardiovascular and thoracic surgeons), diagnostic heart tests (performed by cardiologists), cataract surgery (performed by ophthalmologists), and arthroscopic surgery (performed by orthopedic surgeons).

One potential explanation for this growth is induced demand. Induced demand, however, is generally thought to occur in fields with a large or rapidly increasing number of specialists. The number of specialists practicing in most of these fields did grow, but not nearly as much as utilization did (Roback et al. 1994). As Table 3.3 shows, utilization of these specialty services outpaced supply growth by more than two to one. The long training required to practice in these specialties undoubtedly contributed to the mismatch between supply and demand.[15] Growth in these fields may also have been impeded by medical-specialty boards, which control entry into the specialty fields and can exert cartel power. An increase in the number of specialists practicing in these fields would have *reduced* the growth of individual specialist's incomes.

The importance of changing demand and new skills is also clear in the different experiences of primary-care physicians and specialists over the decade. Primary-care physicians have as much or more opportunity to expand demand (by encouraging visits, for example) as do most specialists. The growth in the primary-care workforce over the 1980s was smaller than the growth in specialty practice (Roback et al. 1994). Nonetheless, primary-care physicians' incomes grew only moderately during the 1980s.

Table 3.3 Growth in procedure utilization, practicing specialists, and specialist incomes for high-income-growth specialties in the United States during the 1980s

Procedure	Increase in utilization	Specialties affected	Change in number of practicing specialists	Increase in income
Coronary artery bypass	174%	Thoracic surgery	−3%	> 100%
Cardiac catheterization	164	Cardiology	61	53
Cataract surgery	123	Ophthalmology	24	43
Hip replacement	72	Orthopedic surgery	37	63

Sources: AMA 1994 (change in number of specialists), DHHS 1993 (coronary artery bypass, cardiac catheterization, hip replacement, and 1980 cataract surgery utilization), Pope and Schneider 1992 (change in incomes, 1983–1988), PROPAC 1993 (1990 cataract surgery).

Note: Figures for coronary artery bypass and cardiac catheterization are based on data for males only. Figures for cataract surgery and hip replacement are based on data for males and females over the age of sixty-five. All figures are for the period 1980–1990 except for increase in income, which are for the period 1983–1988.

Unlike medical specialties, which saw many new techniques and procedures added to the practice of medicine in the 1980s, primary-care practice has remained relatively constant over time. As specialists have proliferated, the complexity of cases seen by general practitioners may have fallen. Patients with serious problems have more opportunities to be referred—or to refer themselves—to specialty care. Many states have changed their laws to permit nurse practitioners and physician assistants to perform some of the functions of primary-care physicians, including prescribing medications. Comparisons of the quality of services provided by these practitioners relative to physicians find that non-physician practitioners perform just as well as doctors for many medical tasks (Sekscenski et al. 1994). Without a change in the demand for their services, and with an increase in the supply of competitors, it is not surprising that the earnings of primary-care physicians remained relatively stable (in real terms) over the decade.

Medicalists are swayed little by the argument that changes in demand and technology generated the increase in specialty incomes that occurred during the 1980s. Some of the increase in the use of these procedures, they argue, was inappropriate, prompted by uninformed consumers and buttressed by the pattern of insurance coverage, since the services of specialists are more likely to be covered by insurance than are those of general practitioners. The lower pay of general practitioners reflects errors in pricing, say the medicalists, not real differences in value. General practitioners in Ontario, Canada, for example, had net incomes as high as those of U.S. general practitioners in 1986; the substantial difference in net earnings between Canadian and U.S. physicians was entirely a product of the much higher earnings of U.S. specialists (GAO 1991).

The rapid rise in specialty earnings and the corresponding increase in practicing specialists have provoked a call for a shift in medical training (and physician reimbursement) away from specialty care and toward primary care. Analysts have come to view the preponderance of specialists among American doctors as a source of inefficiency and cost escalation. In 1961 half of American doctors were generalists, a group defined to include general practitioners, pediatricians, and family practitioners. By 1990 that fraction had fallen below 34 percent. Studies of other countries find current physician mixes much more similar to those of the United States in 1961. Similarly, the ratio of specialists to members in HMOs is lower than the specialist-to-population ratio outside HMOs in the United States (Rivo and Satcher 1993).

Specialists have one to five more years of postgraduate medical training than generalists and earn 50 to 130 percent more annually.[16] Studies find that specialists order more tests and perform more procedures than do general practitioners treating similar disorders (Greenfield et al. 1992). On the basis of these studies, analysts have computed that simply changing the U.S. physician mix back to its 1961 proportions could reduce national health spending by $55 billion in the year 2000, 2 to 5 percent of projected national health spending in that year (Grumbach and Lee 1991).

The starkness of this 1960/1990 comparison, though, obscures the nature of the change over this period. Specialists make up a larger share of the physician population today than they did in 1960, but the number of general practitioners per capita has not declined (Rivo and Satcher 1993). Rather, the increase in the total number of physicians per capita has been an increase in specialists. America may have too many doctors, but, at least by 1960 standards, it does not have too few generalists.

The increasing proportion of American physicians who are specialists is by no means a new phenomenon. Between 1931 and 1949, the share of physicians practicing primary-care medicine dropped from 87 percent to 59 percent (Rivo and Satcher 1993). As early as 1915, a medical reformer complained that patients were bypassing family practitioners and turning directly to specialists; that care was uncoordinated and inefficient (Michael M. Davis, cited in Starr 1982). In 1932 the Committee on the Costs of Medical Care noted that "the incomes of general practitioners and specialists should be more nearly equal than at present" (p. 33). In 1961, when general practitioners made up 50 percent of the physician population, critics complained that the rise of specialization meant that there was no one left to put the "whole man" together again (Somers and Somers 1961). Observers blamed the decline in general practice on the relative lack of status, prestige, and financial rewards reaped by generalists and on the proliferation of insurance for specialty services (Burns 1973; Starr 1982).

While there is a long history of alarm at the rise in specialization, most observers have recognized that specialization is a natural consequence of increased knowledge in medicine—a consequence that follows "modern science as shadow follows substance" (Somers and Somers 1961, p. 29). Such increased specialization is hardly unique to health care. As the amount of information needed to do a job increases in a variety of fields throughout the economy, education levels increase correspondingly. For example, in 1979 a survey of CEOs of the largest U.S. companies found that 68 percent had no degree beyond college. Just nine years later, a second survey found that only 61 percent had no MBA, JD, or alternative higher degree. Surveyors commented that a number of CEOs had both MBAs and JDs (Gentry and Hailey 1980; "Portrait" 1988).[17]

The increased demand for health care, which may in turn be a consequence of increasing medical knowledge, also fed the interest in specialization. As demand for a good grows, the benefits of an increased division of labor also rise—a phenomenon noted by Plato and by Adam Smith. In medicine the increased size of the market means, for example, that there is sufficient demand to support a subspecialist who performs one particular operation exclusively. In turn that subspecialist will become expert in the production of that operation, performing it better and at lower cost than could a generalist. The greater specialization of the physician workforce is more likely a consequence of rising health expenditures than a cause of them.

Within health care, as in other parts of the economy, increasing knowledge and growing markets have overtaken the role of the generalist. In this context, the clamor for more general practitioners may be ill advised. Increases in physician income within specialty and through changes in specialty composition appear to be primarily a response to changes in the demand for particular medical services. The high level of those earnings, though, especially for some specialists, may represent supernormal profits achieved and maintained through the cartel power of specialty boards and of the medical profession in general. The way to reduce those excess individual earnings is to increase the number of specialists, not reduce it.

While increasing the number of specialists would reduce physician incomes, it might lead to an increase in total spending on specialty care. Physicians might induce demand for their services in response to the increased competition, access to specialists would become easier with the increase in supply, and lower prices would draw some patients toward the operating room. Eliminating the cartel could mean that more specialists would be practicing and each individual specialist would earn only a little less. The high earnings of specialists in today's health sector may, perversely, be associated with lower total health care spending.[18]

In any case, a radical change in workforce policy, one that increased the proportion of graduates in primary care to 50 percent, would not have much effect on national health spending for quite some time. Even if medical schools, graduate training programs, and medical students made this initial change, and even if the resulting medical graduates remained in general practice throughout their work lives, by 2020, 25 years after the policy was first implemented, only 42 percent of practicing physicians in the United States would be generalists (Kindig, Cultice, and Mullan 1993). The $55 billion savings from switching to a 1960-style physician composition by 2000 is simply unattainable.[19]

Despite physicians' central role in a system many Americans think fails, most people have high regard for doctors and are quite satisfied with their own (Jacobs, Shapiro, and Schulman 1993). While complaining about medical costs in general, most respondents in one study said that the fee their own physician charged for their most recent visit was appropriate (ibid.). The high incomes earned by physicians appear to reflect primarily a high and growing return related to their skill levels. While these high incomes make a tempting target for revenue raisers, reducing physician incomes alone would not have a significant impact on U.S. health expenditures.

Figure 3.2, which looks at the OECD (excluding the United States), suggests that there is little correlation between physician salary levels and national health expenses as a share of GDP, mainly because physicians' earnings, per se, make up a very small share of total expenses. For this reason, taxing physicians' high earnings, a notion very briefly considered by the Clinton health task force, would have limited effects on health costs. In total, American physicians earned about $100 billion in practice-related income (net of expenses) in 1992.[20] An across-the-board 30 percent net-income tax on physicians would reduce average physician net income levels to their 1980 position. If physicians did not change their practice patterns in any way, though, this rather sweeping cost cut would reduce the level of national health spending by only 3.5 percent, less than one year's worth of cost growth.[21]

If reducing doctors' incomes led to certain kinds of changes in physician practice, such as fewer surgical procedures and diagnostic tests,

Health spending/GDP

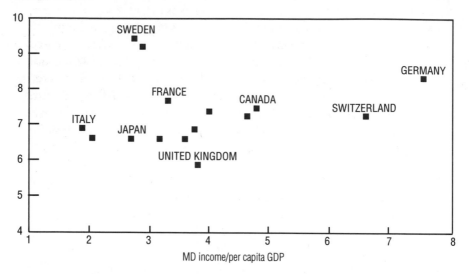

MD income/per capita GDP

Figure 3.2   Relative income of physicians and OECD health spending as a share of GDP, 1980. All OECD nations with per capita income of more than $2,500 in 1980 other than the United States are included, with selected countries labeled. (*Source:* OECD 1993b.)

costs would be reduced further. Of course, some of these tests are un-necessary. But across-the-board income cuts would almost certainly lead as well to reductions in the number of valuable tests and proce-dures, and to reductions in the length of physician visits—changes that would surely diminish the quality of medical care. Changes in the com-position of the physician workforce might reduce spending more, but such changes would take a long time to have effects. Furthermore, shifting the composition of the workforce toward generalists would move medicine in the opposite direction from the patterns observed in the remainder of the economy—reducing, rather than raising, skill lev-els in the face of an explosion of information.

Variations in Utilization

Medicalists point to large variations in health care utilization as evidence that significant savings could be squeezed out of the system through scientific rationalization. A related source of potential savings comes from the elimination of procedures that are inappropriate. Concern about appropriateness arises from studies of patterns in the use of medical procedures that find huge variations in their use across small areas—variations that cannot be explained by simple demographic characteristics of the underlying population. In 1969, for example, the use of tonsillectomies was over ten times higher in some counties in Vermont than in similar neighboring counties. Even the use of such well-established surgical procedures as appendectomies varies significantly among areas of the United States (Wennberg and Gittelsohn 1973).

Tenfold variations in the use of procedures strongly hint that someone is doing something wrong. Either high-utilization areas egregiously overuse medical services or low-utilization areas neglect promising treatments. But this is nothing new. The authors of studies of variations in hospital use in the 1930s were troubled by their implications: if medicine is truly scientific, they believed, there "ought to be norms" for service provision (Stevens 1989). A growing interest in the appropriateness of care has emerged from the evidence on variations in utilization. As one contemporary critic notes, "The implication [of variation studies] . . . is that medical resources are almost certainly used inefficiently. That is . . . , medical benefits per dollar spent could be significantly increased" (Aaron 1991, p. 21).

Most variation studies do not distinguish between valuable and nonvaluable care. A few recent studies, though, have examined records to determine whether practice patterns are, using medical criteria, "appropriate." In most such studies, the term is defined so that for a patient with a particular condition, a procedure is appropriate if the probability that it will be medically effective exceeds the danger it poses. These studies have found, based on medical-record reviews, that some 32 percent of carotid endarterectomies, 14 percent of coronary artery bypass surgeries, and 20 percent of pacemaker insertions were inappropriately performed (Leape 1989). In the endarterectomy and bypass studies, an additional 30 to 32 percent of procedures were rated as of equivocal value.

These figures are alarming. Many Americans are receiving treatments that experts rate as providing them with no benefits, and that may well harm them. Furthermore, the procedures identified as having high rates of inappropriateness are both costly and frequently performed. In 1986 hospital costs were $8,600 for an endarterectomy, $24,000 for a coronary artery bypass graft (CABG), and $12,500 for a pacemaker implantation (Lemrow et al. 1990). Looking at these three procedures alone, simply not doing those that were inappropriate or equivocal would have improved Americans' health and saved close to $4 billion in 1986.[22]

While studies have succeeded in documenting variations both in practice patterns and in the appropriateness of practices, researchers have failed to identify consistent relationships between these two kinds of variation. Many, though not all, studies show that areas with more beds and physicians generally utilize services more than do those with fewer facilities (Leape 1989). But further evidence suggests that the variations result is not a consequence of doctors and hospitals in areas with more competition inducing demand for unnecessary services.

Consider the evidence from a group of patients who might be expected to be impervious to the importuning of physicians: members of physicians' families. Physicians' families face very low charges for medical interventions and might be expected to use more medical services because physicians typically do not charge one another for services rendered. Even compared with well-insured nonphysicians, however, physicians' families use more interventions (Leape 1989). Since physicians are not compensated for these procedures and physicians' family members are much better informed about their efficacy than the lay public, the high rates of use in physicians' families cannot be explained by an exploitation hypothesis. Instead, it seems likely that physicians' families simply have a preference for more procedures.

A few recent appropriateness studies directly examine the relationship between inappropriate utilization and high utilization. Surprisingly, these studies find that the proportion of procedures that are inappropriate is unrelated to the number of procedures that are performed (Chassin et al. 1987; McGlynn et al. 1994). One recent study compared the use of coronary artery bypass surgery in New York State and in Ontario using both American and Canadian appropriateness criteria. Overall, the rate of bypass surgery is about 40 percent higher in New York State than in Ontario (Anderson et al. 1993). While a greater number of cases in both countries were ranked inappropriate using Canadian criteria as opposed to U.S. criteria, the rates of inappropriate care were virtually identical in both countries under both sets of criteria (McGlynn et al. 1994). Residents of high-utilization areas undergo more inappropriate procedures than do residents of low-utilization areas, but they also experience more appropriate procedures.[23] Conversely, residents of low-utilization areas have fewer appropriate procedures as well as fewer inappropriate procedures. In low-utilization areas, some people who would have been appropriately treated had they sought care in high-utilization areas will not receive treatment.

Appropriateness studies to date have not examined the appropriateness of not performing a given procedure. Just as some procedures may be inappropriately performed (errors of commission), others may be inappropriately neglected (errors of omission). The significant variations in the use of procedures whose efficacy is documented suggest skepticism about the potential total dollar savings from reducing inappropriate utilization. Clearly, reducing inappropriate use and nonuse of procedures would improve Americans' health, but the effect on total spending will depend on the balance between the current level of inappropriate use and inappropriate nonuse.

If variations do not arise because of greed, why do they occur? Some evidence suggests that variations stem from uncertainty about appropriate practice (Leape 1989). Physicians treat in accordance with the methods they learned from their mentors in medical school and residency programs and from what they observe their peers doing. The enormous scientific uncertainty with respect to most medical practices makes it possible for well-trained, respected, honest physicians to differ radically in their prescriptions for treatment. These honest differences of opinion, communicated to medical-school students and local peers, generate regional variations in treatment patterns.

Evidence of such uncertainty is widespread (Eddy 1984). In studies of preferred treatment in hypothetical cases, physicians' opinions about appropriate care run the gamut from watchful waiting to radical intervention. Panels convened to recommend guidelines for the assessment of appropriate use often classify an enormous fraction (up to half) of cases in the equivocal category (Leape 1989). Some equivocal cases may lie on the borderline between situations in which treatments are known to be effective and those in which they are known to be ineffective. Most, though, are situations for which firm evidence on efficacy (or inefficacy) is simply not available.

Properly executed clinical trial studies are the gold standard in measuring appropriateness. These very costly and lengthy studies provide accurate information about the efficacy of a given treatment by comparing patients randomly assigned to treatment with similar patients randomly selected to receive a placebo. Such trials, however, have been completed for only a tiny fraction of the procedures available to physicians. The Institute of Medicine (1985) estimates that fewer than 20 percent of medical interventions have been properly tested in a clinical trial.

Every reform proposal stresses the importance of developing treatment guidelines based on clinical trials to reduce the enormous uncertainty that exists in medical practice. Unfortunately, the cost (in time and money) of effectiveness studies is so great that any development of guidelines will likely be overwhelmed by the number of new innovations introduced. Simply developing the *criteria* for guidelines costs $0.5 million to $1 million per procedure (Brook and McGlynn 1994). Furthermore, variations persist even where guidelines exist (Leape 1989). Communicating results to physicians requires substantial effort. Managed-care and utilization review organizations would seem to have some clout to enforce treatment guidelines. To date, however, they have not proved very effective in doing so.

Even randomized trials provide only an indicator of appropriateness in a particular case. The trials typically enroll a very narrowly defined sample of patients with uncomplicated conditions. Participating physicians are drawn from the top ranks of academic medicine. But the cases that are seen in ordinary practice are likely to fall outside the range of patients who were studied in the trial. As physicians grow more comfortable with a procedure, they are likely to extend its use to patients with more complications—patients for whom the clinical trial results may or may not apply.

Consider the case of coronary artery bypass surgery. Early trials of this procedure examined a selected group of patients under age sixty-five (almost all men) and found benefits for some categories of patient (Leape et al. 1991). In 1973, 90 percent of the patients undergoing this surgery were, like those in the trials, under sixty-five, although this group likely included many patients with other conditions besides blocked arteries and with more complications than those in the randomized trials. By 1991, though, almost half the patients undergoing this surgery were over sixty-five (DHHS 1993). Only a small minority fit into the demographic and clinical categories of patients examined in the original trials, but no further large randomized trials have been completed. A similar pattern occurred for angioplasty. Initially, studies suggested that patients under sixty would benefit. As surgeons tried the procedure on older patients, they began to believe that these patients would benefit too (Hilborne et al. 1991).

Evidence from practice supports this conjecture in both cases. The mortality rate of patients who undergo CABG surgery has declined significantly over time, even as the patients having the surgery have been sicker and older (Leape et al. 1991). Recent evidence suggest that patients aged eighty to ninety-two have results from angioplasty almost as good as those of the population under sixty (Hilborne et al. 1991). The extension of these procedures to older populations was not directly supported by randomized clinical trials, but it may have been appropriate.

The relationship between experience and effectiveness further complicates that between appropriateness and variations. Considerable evidence—and common sense—suggest that as doctors gain experience with a procedure they become better at doing it (Hood, Scott, and Evoy 1984; Leape et al. 1991). A procedure that would have been very dangerous if performed by a newly trained physician in 1980 may prove beneficial when performed by a very experienced physician ten years later. In areas where physicians use a procedure more frequently, the threshold for appropriateness may be lower. In areas where physicians, hospitals, and nurses have little experience with a procedure, simple cases may be inappropriate, while in other areas complex procedures may be appropriate.

Finally, certain variations in medical practice stem from differences in patient preferences. Although variation studies typically examine the use of costly, complex, and well-reported surgical and diagnostic procedures, variations of similar magnitude also exist in the use of less costly primary-care procedures. Dental visits per capita, for example, are 33 percent more frequent in the West of the United States than in the South (DHHS 1993). Even variations in common surgical procedures are affected by differences in patient preferences. For example, much of the variation in the use of cataract surgery stems from differences in the frequency of patients complaining about vision problems to their physicians (Escarce 1993).

The role of patient preferences in variations is likely to grow as patients become better informed about surgical procedures. Recent studies of prostate surgery, for example, found significant variations in the willingness of patients with similar medical conditions to undergo surgery after being presented with complete information on the risks and benefits of the procedure (Kasper, Mulley, and Wennberg 1992). Such variations reflect differences in underlying patient preferences about states of health and illness and in attitudes toward doctors, hospitals, and medical treatment. These preferences may be concentrated in particular communities. Residents of Hawaii are three times more likely to wear their seat belts when driving than are residents of Rhode Island (Department of Transportation 1991). Residents of Utah are half as likely to smoke as are residents of West Virginia or Nevada (Van Son 1993).

While the use of guidelines may make physician practices more uniform, the expansion of efforts to inform patients about health benefits and risks may instead lead to increases in practice variations. Improved information could reduce the dollar costs of medical care (if better-informed patients reject procedures more frequently) or could increase costs (if better-informed patients choose more treatment). Whether reducing variations raises or lowers national health spending, though, improving physician and patient information will undoubtedly increase the benefits per dollar spent on medical care.

Moral Hazard

Medicalists believe that the best way to save money in the health sector is by changing the roles and behaviors of those who provide and administer health care—doctors, hospitals, and insurers. But marketists argue that savings might be more successfully achieved by changing the behavior of consumers. American consumers pay a smaller share of health bills out of their own pockets today than ever in the past. The fact that someone else is paying for their health bills undoubtedly makes them use health services that they would not use otherwise.

Between 1960 and 1990, the share of health care payments made out-of-pocket declined from 50 percent to 20 percent (Levit et al. 1994). This decline had a substantial effect on health spending. In the RAND health insurance experiment, a controlled study conducted in the late 1970s, people who paid none of their medical expenses out-of-pocket consumed about 40 percent more medical services than did those who had to pay the first $1,000 of their expenses out-of-pocket (Newhouse 1993a). Based on such measurements of the effect of declines in out-of-pocket spending on the use of health services, it can be estimated that the declining share of out-of-pocket payments alone would have led to an increase in real national health expenditures between 1960 and 1990 of almost $70 billion (my calculation, based on data in Newhouse 1992b).

Out-of-pocket health spending declined as both public and private health insurance expanded in the United States over these decades. People with insurance pay up front for a policy that shoulders some of the financial burden if an untoward event occurs in the future. In effect, insurance reduces the price of insured events.

Insurance beneficiaries tend to respond to this decline in the price of insured events by scaling back their efforts to minimize these costs, either by reducing the precautions they take to avoid undesired events or by spending more when such events occur. This reduction in price means that people with insurance are more likely than the uninsured to leave their car doors unlocked, to purchase costly jewelry, or to build their homes in hurricane zones. In the extreme, some people with insurance may even burn down their own homes to collect insurance money. This response to insurance is known in the economics literature as "moral hazard."

In the case of health care, people with insurance coverage may take more health risks than those without coverage (for example, they might be more likely to indulge in risky sports activities). People with health insurance also have less incentive to minimize the cost of the care they use after they become ill. In auto and home ownership insurance contracts, payments by insurers depend on the initial value of the good insured; policyholders have no incentive to seek additional or more costly repair services. But a policyholder who becomes ill collects no benefits from the insurance company (in these contracts) unless he or she sees a doctor; the total payment made by the insurance company depends entirely on the number of procedures the individual chooses to undergo. This kind of open-ended insurance contract makes the moral-hazard problems that arise after an illness has developed more important in health care than in auto or home insurance. Insured people go to doctors much more often than uninsured people; they may also be more likely to see particularly costly doctors and specialists (although there is no evidence of such behavior in the RAND health insurance experiment; Manning et al. 1987). The moral hazard that accompanies insurance is what leads policymakers to believe that extending coverage will increase the use of health services by the poor. Without moral hazard, insurance would simply redistribute income, without increasing the use of services.

The reason moral hazard is a problem is that someone must pay for these higher levels of use. Insurers must recoup the costs of their payments through higher premiums. Ultimately, these higher payments reduce the welfare of those insured. To see how this works, suppose you have a really severe headache. Without insurance, you might take two aspirin and wait until tomorrow. With full insurance, you might insist on seeing a doctor, perhaps even a specialist, who might order a magnetic-resonance-imaging (MRI) scan to ensure that your problem is not a brain tumor and, upon learning that it is not, send you home to take two aspirins. The health outcome is the same, but with the MRI scan, the outcome comes at a much higher cost. The cost of your MRI scan will be spread among all premium payers, so you will pay only a small fraction of the cost you yourself incurred. But if the insurance company cannot monitor behavior at all, it will eventually raise your premium to reflect the heavier patterns of use of MRI scans by you and all other insured people who behave like you. Eventually, you and other consumers will pay the full cost of the additional MRI scans through higher insurance premiums. This increase in premium will occur despite the likelihood that given the choice between buying expensive coverage that explicitly pays for the cost of an MRI scan and buying less costly coverage that forces you to wait a day, you would have chosen the wait-a-day policy.

As this example illustrates, moral hazard occurs because insurance companies cannot fully monitor the behavior of those they insure. If your insurance company could monitor the severity of your headache, it could make a deal with you. In exchange for restrictions on your ability to get a reimbursable MRI scan, it could charge you a lower premium. You might well prefer this deal to the alternative of paying higher premiums in exchange for no restrictions on your choices. Insurers are increasingly using monitoring to reduce the cost of moral hazard. Monitoring takes the form of utilization review requirements, second-opinion requirements, and health maintenance organizations that limit the resources available to the insured. Other insurers pay doctors on a capitation, or per-patient basis, and hospitals on a diagnosis-related flat-fee basis, known as DRG. These forms of payment do not increase insurer payouts according to how many services a patient uses. Instead, both give providers incentives to limit care.

Insurance contracts that do not fully monitor behavior typically contain financial incentives to reduce moral hazard, in the form of consumer out-of-pocket payments called copayments and deductibles. These features of contracts are designed to leave policyholders with incentives to avoid accidents and to minimize at least the initial costs of accidents. In health insurance, the most common nonmonitored contracts limit the potential out-of-pocket payments that may be made by a policyholder to about $1,000.[24] Above this limit, there are no monetary incentives within such insurance contracts to reduce the use of costly services.

The public-policy importance of health care and the existence of experimental evidence on the magnitude of moral hazard associated with health insurance have focused attention on the role of moral hazard-inducing insurance in driving up health costs. But developed economies are characterized by high levels of insurance in all sectors and in most of these sectors moral hazard does not seem to result in the runaway costs observed in health care. In the United States, the property and casualty insurance market collected $223 billion in premiums in 1991 (Galt 1994) and life insurers collected an additional $79 billion for their products (American Council of Life Insurers 1993). Nor are other sectors immune to moral hazard. Because of moral hazard, insurance increases the likelihood of house-destroying fires and automobile-destroying collisions. It raises the probability that insured motion pictures will be delayed during production and that companies who purchase patent infringement insurance will encroach on the research of others. In some sectors moral hazard may be quantitatively quite important. For example, the property and casualty insurance industry estimates that more than 20 percent of nonresidential fires are suspicious in origin (Insurance Information Institute 1990). Despite the pervasiveness of insurance and the importance of moral hazard, these sectors have had much more stable costs than has health care. Insurance alone cannot be the explanation for cost growth in the health sector.

One might expect the role of moral hazard in health insurance to be quantitatively smaller than in many other kinds of insurance. The non-monetary, noninsurable costs—pain, suffering, and time—associated with becoming ill and using many medical services are high enough to act as a significant deterrent to overuse of health care services. In fact, the decreasing share of U.S. medical expenses that are paid out-of-pocket cannot explain much of the change in total health spending. The higher share of health care costs covered by insurance in 1990 as compared with 1960 appears to have accounted for a $70 billion increase in health care spending; but the total increase in those three decades was over $600 billion. The spread of insurance was thus responsible for only about one-tenth of the actual rise in spending (Newhouse 1993a).

Moral Hazard and Spending Growth

Analyses of moral hazard usually focus on increases in spending at a point in time. The puzzle in health care, though, concerns the rate of growth in spending over time. Conventional moral-hazard stories do not explain the high rate of growth in health spending at all. To address this problem, some analysts have postulated that moral hazard and the development of new medical technologies can interact in a way that adds a dynamic dimension to the problems associated with insurance.

In these models, insurance expands the market for new treatment technologies and encourages their development. Because of the moral hazard in insurance contracts, policyholders will use new treatments—for example, less painful diagnostic testing—that they do not fully value. Technology developers, in turn, will respond by overinvesting in the development of these technologies. Such moral hazard-induced technological development could, in theory, actually make people worse off, if it leads to the production of technologies that, absent moral hazard, consumers would not choose to purchase (or to cover in their insurance contracts). Unless insurers can observe whether those purchasing a technology truly value it, they must raise their premiums to cover the cost of the technology for both those who fully value it and those who purchase it only because of moral hazard. Some people, though, would prefer not to have access to the technology rather than pay the full price for it (Goddeeris 1984; Weisbrod 1991). If insurers cannot monitor the use of services, these people will not be able to buy low-cost contracts that exclude these less highly valued technologies.

Although the possibility of excessive technological development spurred by moral hazard exists in principle, whether such development occurs depends on the difficulty of writing good insurance contracts, on the nature of technological change, and on the form of these contracts (Baumgardner 1991). Utilization review, managed care, and higher copayment rates should be able to reduce the technology-related inefficiencies induced by insurance in the long run, just as they do in the case of moral hazard at a point in time. A range of empirical evidence, though, suggests that health costs have also risen quickly under more restrictive contracts. HMOs, for example, typically offer much the same package of technologies as fee-for-service plans. Until recently, costs in HMOs grew as quickly as those in fee-for-service plans in the United States (Schwartz 1987; Newhouse 1992a). Similarly, rates of cost growth in other countries, where the supply of medical technologies is centrally controlled, have been quite similar to those in the United States (Newhouse 1992b). As I discuss in Chapter 4, cost growth was also very rapid before health insurance became widespread, and cost growth in uninsured sectors of health care has been almost as rapid as in well-insured sectors.

Moral Hazard, the Tax Treatment of Insurance, and Catastrophic Health Care Coverage

Imperfectly monitored insurance provides benefits, in the form of protection from risks, but has costs, in the form of increased moral hazard. Consumers trade off the diminished risk for the increased cost, in health insurance as in other areas of insurance. Simulation estimates suggest that for the average consumer, the best trade-off involves coinsurance rates considerably higher than those that currently prevail (Feldstein 1973; Feldman and Dowd 1991). These estimates suggest that consumers would be better off with a policy providing for 95 percent copayments up to $1,000 (in late-1970s dollars) rather than a free-care or less-than-95-percent coinsurance policy. The 25-percent-coinsurance-level policy used in the RAND health insurance experiment most closely approximates average health insurance today. Moving from that policy to a 95-percent-copayment policy would, according to these calculations, improve consumer welfare (because consumers would save money in exchange for giving up services they do not value highly). It would also reduce national health spending by 10 to 15 percent.[25] Some analysts assert that excessive insurance also leads to increases in the price and quality of health care that would not have been captured by the RAND experiment (Feldstein 1973). If that is the case, savings from higher coinsurance policies could be even greater.

If consumers would be better off buying higher-coinsurance policies, why don't they do so? Marketists argue that in the case of health insurance, the trade-off between moral hazard and risk bearing is distorted by tax policy. The tax subsidy for health insurance may induce people to choose more risk protection and higher costs than they would otherwise select.

Health insurance payments made by an employer on behalf of an employee are treated for tax purposes as a business expense for the employer, but they are not treated as taxable income to the employee. An employee who receives a one-dollar increase in wages must pay a substantial proportion of this increase to the government as taxes. When the same employee instead receives a health insurance policy that costs his employer one dollar more to provide, none of this increase in payments must be paid as taxes.

The effect of this tax exemption is to give a worker a discount on the purchase of health insurance equal to his or her marginal tax rate. The discount encourages people to demand more insurance coverage through their employers than they would if they had to pay full price. These exemptions apply only to benefits purchased through employers. Individuals who purchase health insurance benefits on their own face the full cost of the purchase. In 1993 marginal federal tax rates for the median family were 26 percent, including social security taxes (CBO 1994d). State income-tax rates ranged between 0 and 12 percent, so the total discount on health insurance premiums for the median family was between 26 and 38 percent (CEA 1993). When increases in premiums are discounted at almost 40 percent, there is less reason to purchase contracts that minimize moral hazard.

The employment-based nature of the tax subsidy generates signifi-

cant distortions in the health insurance market. By encouraging employment-based purchase only, the tax subsidy hurts people who would
be better off buying insurance on their own, particularly young people
who frequently change jobs (Glied 1994). It should be eliminated. But
empirical estimates suggest that the tax exemption for employer-provided health insurance has relatively little effect on total health spending. It may raise total health costs by 5 to 15 percent (Chernick, Holmer, and Weinberg 1987; CBO 1994d). Eliminating the benefit would
save money, but mainly by leading people to drop insurance altogether.
Only 5 to 7 percent could be saved through people buying less coverage.[26]

Although catastrophic plans, with very high deductibles, are offered
by many indemnity health insurers, few Americans purchase them. Even
among those who purchased nongroup coverage (receiving no tax subsidy and paying higher insurance rates), a majority in 1977 bought
policies with low or standard deductibles (under $100 in 1977; Farley
1986). The existence of a safety net that provides free care in emer-
gencies to people who lack substantial income or health insurance reduces the appeal of high-deductible coverage to low-income people
who might otherwise be tempted by its low premiums. Conventional
wisdom among insurers is that most Americans who do choose catastrophic plans already have coverage through a spouse and use the catastrophic plan only as backup coverage. This lack of interest in catastrophic coverage was noted as far back as 1953 (Serbein 1953).

In the RAND health insurance experiment, people who had been assigned to high-coinsurance (catastrophic-style) plans were asked whether
they would purchase supplemental coverage to reduce their cost sharing
if they were offered such plans. Forty percent of those in the high-
coinsurance plans said they would have purchased full supplementation
if it had been offered; all but 23 percent would have purchased at least
partial supplementation (Newhouse 1993a). In the 1980s, as concern
over health costs increased, enrollment in plans with higher deductibles
did grow. Deductibles in nonmanaged-care plans covering one person
rose from an average of $172 in 1988 to $223 in 1993 (Gabel et al.
1994). This 30 percent increase, however, just traced the increase in
real per capita spending over this period. The average coinsurance rate,
measured by the share of payments made out-of-pocket, continued to
decline.

Very tightly monitored forms of insurance coverage, such as closed-panel health maintenance organizations, can reduce health spending (by limiting utilization) about as much as high-deductible fee-for-service policies (Newhouse 1993b). In recent years many purchasers have chosen to reduce their premiums by buying coverage with more limitations on utilization. Growth in managed-care membership, though, has occurred mainly in plans offering flexible packages that permit subscribers to seek care outside the plan (albeit at a higher price). These preferred-provider and point-of-service plans have grown explosively. PPO membership grew from 28 million in 1987 to 85 million in 1991. Together, PPOs and point-of-service plans now command almost one-quarter of the employer-based health insurance market, a larger share than is held by traditional HMOs (HIAA 1992). Apparently, Americans are more willing to accept policies with substantial insurer oversight than they are those with high deductibles, but even insurer oversight is not readily accepted.

The desire to buy complete coverage, despite the moral-hazard penalty, is prevalent in other kinds of consumer insurance as well. While insurance with a very high deductible is usually much less costly than insurance without such a deductible, the most popular auto collision and comprehensive policies include only limited up-front deductibles. Among purchasers of comprehensive auto insurance coverage from one very large New York State insurer in 1992, for example, 23 percent bought the most generous policies, which have no deductible for broken window glass and only a $50 deductible on other damage.[27] By contrast, 28 percent bought coverage with a general deductible of $500 or more, though even in this group, most chose no deductible on window glass (New York State 1995).[28]

People may choose these plans because they are willing to pay a lot to avoid financial risk. They may also buy low-deductible coverage because they do not want to consider price when a problem occurs (Vladeck 1981; Fuchs 1986). Consumers may recognize that at the point that they need to choose a service a substantial deductible will discourage use. If, however, they believe that such use would be a long-term benefit to them, they might want to eliminate price from their decision to use services when they become ill (Thaler and Shefrin 1981). The persistence of ill health may further discourage the purchase of high-deductible coverage, especially if it is difficult to switch coverage from year to year. Consumers who are ill this year are also likely to have higher-than-average expenditures next year, and this increases the financial risks associated with high-deductible coverage (Zook, Moore, and Zeckhauser 1981).

Finally, noneconomists may view health insurance as something other than a true insurance contract. This difference in views became evident during the design of the benefit package for the Clinton Health Security Act. The health care task force considered a number of benefit packages, among them a Blue Cross standard package and a catastrophic coverage plan, with a $2,000 deductible, that could be mandated for firms that had not previously offered insurance and enriched over time.

The two packages were debated in a meeting before the president and cabinet. Two teams, each including financial and political analysts, presented the two sides of the debate. The catastrophic team showed that financial savings under catastrophic coverage would be substantial, with deficit reduction possible almost immediately. But the standard-benefit team won with a simple argument: fewer than 20 percent of Americans would actually receive a cash benefit under the mandated catastrophic-insurance policy in a given year.[29] The rest would spend less than $2,000.

The economists at the meeting were startled. To economists, insurance protects against risky events. People with home insurance benefit from the security of the policy, knowing that if their house burns down they will be protected. They do not benefit any less from owning home insurance because their house does not burn down. Non-economists, though, frequently assert that it was a waste of money to buy an insurance policy that they never "used." To non-economists, health insurance is not entirely about risk; it is also a form of prepayment for services. This difference in viewpoint helps explain why, as one commentator flatly put it, "there is no political support for cost containment based on requiring substantial patient cost sharing" (Berenson 1994, p. 186).

Whatever the reason that people choose relatively complete and un-monitored insurance, health planners cannot ignore this preference. That is not to say that the preference should be mandated or encouraged. Tax policy that encourages people to buy health insurance protection that they do not value at its full cost wastes public funds. And some people (especially economists) do buy insurance policies with substantial deductibles. Nonetheless, reform policies that depend on large numbers of people choosing insurance with significant deductibles or very comprehensive monitoring are unlikely to achieve their results. The tax subsidy estimates suggest that imposing a 30 to 40 percent tax penalty on the purchase of additional dollars of health insurance coverage would induce Americans to reduce spending voluntarily by only 5 to 15 percent, the equivalent of less than two years of real-cost growth. Furthermore, the evidence suggests that reducing insurance would have limited effects on the long-run growth rate of health spending.

How Much Could Be Saved?

Overall, the evidence suggests that only limited, onetime savings can be achieved through onetime reductions in health costs. Curtailing moral hazard by completely eliminating the tax subsidy to health insurance might save as much as 15 percent of national health costs, a little more than two years' worth of real-cost growth. Slashing administrative costs could save, in the most optimistic scenario, less than 9 percent of national health costs, which is less than two years' worth of cost growth. Eliminating all malpractice costs and defensive medicine could save 4.5 percent of national health costs, or less than the difference in costs between 1990 and 1991. Reducing physician incomes to 1980 levels would yield one-half year's worth of savings. Attenuating inappropriate use of medical procedures might save more, but to the extent that a program to uncover excess usage might also reveal underutilized procedures, the effects on spending (though not on health) are equivocal.

Any attempt to cut costs substantially, even once, would require a drastic overhaul of the health sector and would yield only limited savings. It would be virtually impossible to achieve the maximum savings from all these strategies at once because they employ conflicting methods of cost control. For example, a system that eliminated coinsurance would reduce administrative costs but would increase moral hazard. Nonetheless, even if it were possible, the sum of these effects would reduce national health spending by only 33 percent—from the 1993 level back to the 1986 level. Furthermore, most of these changes would have other negative repercussions. Cutting administrative costs would make it harder for the system to absorb new information. Reducing malpractice costs would leave people uncompensated for their injuries. Curtailing physician incomes would change the nature of physician practice in ways that might reduce the quality of care.

The overwhelming role of cost growth in the health cost equation can be seen in a comparison of U.S. and Canadian health costs. U.S. per capita health care costs in 1985 were about $2,000 and Canadian costs were $1,550. Suppose that the U.S. government had waved a magic wand in 1985 and reduced national per capita health care costs to the Canadian level. At current rates of cost growth, U.S. costs would still be back up to $2,000 by 1990. This apparently bold experiment would have bought only five years of health-care-cost respite.[30]

The magnitude of health expenditures is so large that savings from efficiency improvements would fund many important programs and projects. But they would not solve the underlying problem. These one-time savings would rapidly be swamped by continuing cost growth.

4 ///

Can We Afford
More Health Care?

In December 1992, just before taking office, President Clinton declared that something had to be done about health care; otherwise, he said emphatically, "It's going to bankrupt this country" (Friedman 1992). Many Americans, including the president and members of Congress from both parties, believe health care in the United States is just too expensive. Health care now comprises almost 14 percent of the value of all goods and services produced in the United States (Levit et al. 1994). Other developed countries spend far less. In 1990 average per capita spending in the next-most-costly country, Canada, was 30 percent lower than in the United States; Germany spent half as much per capita as the United States; the United Kingdom spent only 35 percent as much (CBO 1993c). Not only are American costs high today, but they are growing fast. Analysts project that by 2020, the health care sector will consume more than one-quarter of the GDP (Burner, Waldo, and McKusick 1992).

Neither high nor rising costs are news to the U.S. health care system. Costs have been growing faster than overall inflation since at least 1935, and probably earlier. The Committee on the Costs of Medical Care (1932) remarked in passing that health care costs had had and would continue to have a tendency to rise as medicine progressed.

While the United States has always been among the highest spenders and spends much more on health care today than other countries do, the rate of growth in per capita health spending has been remarkably similar in developed countries that operate very different health care systems.[1] Over the past few decades, the annual rate of increase in real per capita health care costs in the OECD countries ranged between 3 and 9 percent (see Figure 4.1). The U.S. rate of 4.9 percent per year was the tenth lowest among the 24 OECD nations. Over the more recent 1985–1993 period, U.S. cost growth ranked seventh highest among the OECD nations.

The main effect of changes in health policy on spending has involved where the bills for rising health costs get paid. The share of health care expenditures paid directly out-of-pocket by consumers has fallen steadily as a share of total expenditures. In 1960 Americans paid more than one-half of their health bills directly; by the late 1980s, more than three-fourths of costs were paid through private and public insurance, mainly financed through employer-paid premiums and taxes. As a consequence of these changes, costs for the nation as a whole have grown rapidly, while direct costs to consumers have changed very little. Even

Growth rate (%)

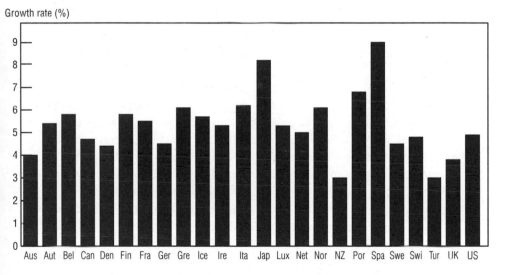

Figure 4.1 The growth of health spending in the OECD over three decades. Growth rates shown are the real per capita rate for each nation adjusted by its GDP deflator. Data for Luxembourg and Portugal are for the years 1970 to 1990. Data for Turkey are for the years 1975 to 1990. Data for all other nations are for the years 1960 to 1990.

during the 1980s, when workers complained that firms were reducing the generosity of coverage, the share of expenses paid out-of-pocket fell by 4 percent (Letsch et al. 1992). Indeed, the share of health expenditures paid out-of-pocket in the United States is smaller than the share of costs not covered by public insurance in 13 of the 23 other OECD nations.[2]

The declining out-of-pocket share of expenditures has deflected the rise in costs away from consumers. Although health care costs have risen rapidly as a share of national income, they have risen little as a share of personal income. In 1989 direct health care costs (including out-of-pocket payments for services and consumer premium contributions) comprised a smaller share of personal after-tax income than they had in 1972 (Levit and Cowan 1991).[3]

U.S. workers today pay for health care before, not after, they receive their paychecks. Most of the burden of increasing private costs has been borne by workers through increased health costs in business payrolls. The share of expenditures paid by business insurance plans rose from 16 percent in 1965 to 28 percent in 1991. Business insurance costs make up part of the total cost of labor compensation. The share of employee compensation that went to pay health insurance premiums more than tripled between 1965 and 1990—from 1.8 percent of compensation in 1965 to 7.6 percent in 1991 (Cowan and McDonnell 1993).

The increase in health care costs has also fallen heavily on all levels of government. Rising health costs cripple efforts to limit government spending. Health care accounted for only 11.6 percent of federal expenditures in 1980, but it had reached 20 percent of federal expenditures in 1994 and—if no changes are made—was projected to consume as much as 33 percent of the federal budget by 2004 (CBO 1994a). Simply limiting the rate of growth in federal health care spending to the rate of growth in GDP would cut the projected year 2004 deficit by 80 percent.[4] At the state and local government level, health care spending is projected to be almost 2.5 times higher in 2000 than it was in 1991 (CBO 1992).

The Inexorable Rise in Health Care Spending

In the United States, the rapid rate of growth in health costs has already persisted through a variety of formidable changes in the economy and in the health system. In the 1920s, before the advent of health insurance, hospitals competed by offering ever more luxurious services and surroundings, and increasingly specialized equipment, much as they do today. The real value of hospital construction in the late 1920s amounted to $7.5 billion (in 1993 dollars; Stevens 1989), about the same share of the GDP at the time as health facilities construction comprises today. As Table 4.1 shows, hospital costs continued to grow rapidly through the worst of the Great Depression. From 1935 through 1940, a period when almost all health costs were paid out-of-pocket, per capita expenditures grew at a rate of 4.7 percent a year (after accounting for economy-wide inflation). Per capita cost growth marched onward at a very similar pace through the subsequent decades, despite massive institutional changes. Per capita costs grew faster than per capita GDP through the 1940s and 1950s, as private insurance spread. They grew faster than GDP in the 1960s, through the introduction of Medicare and Medicaid, and they grew faster than GDP in the 1970s and 1980s as the government tried to rein in the growth of both programs. Most forecasters, sensibly basing their predictions on past experience, project that health care costs will continue to grow at similar

Table 4.1 Rates of growth in per capita health spending, hospital costs, and GDP, and percentage with hospital insurance at end of period

Time period	All health spending (annual growth rate)[a]	Hospital costs (annual growth rate)[a]	GDP (annual growth rate)[b]	Percentage with hospital insurance at end of period
1929–1935	−0.29%	5.41%	−3.82%	< 6%
1935–1940	4.65	4.53	5.07	9
1940–1950	4.62	6.77	3.14	51
1950–1960	4.04	4.92	1.57	72
1960–1970	6.22	7.31	2.56	> 86
1970–1980	3.82	4.68	1.85	> 86
1980–1990	4.41	3.69	1.63	> 86

Sources: Health spending, hospital cost, and GDP data are from Department of Commerce 1975 (for 1929 through 1960) and Letsch et al. 1992 (for 1961 through 1990). Hospital insurance data are from Department of Commerce 1975 (for 1929 through 1960, private insurance only) and HIAA 1993 (for 1961 through 1990, government-provided and private insurance).
   a. Deflated by the Consumer Price Index.
   b. Adjusted by the GDP deflator.

rates, reaching 18 percent of GDP by the year 2000 and 32 percent by 2030 (Burner et al. 1992).

Costs have also grown rapidly in sectors of the health care market where concerns about insurance, the value of life, administrative intrusiveness, and the government's role are less important. Consider veterinary medicine, for example. Very few Americans purchase veterinary insurance to cover their dogs and cats and most are willing to euthanatize a sick pet, so concerns about the high costs of prolonging the life of very sick patients do not come into play. Nonetheless, costs in veterinary medicine have increased as the technology of pet care has improved. Veterinary expenditures for dogs and cats rose from $4 billion in 1987 to almost $7 billion in 1991, an increase of more than 40 percent in constant dollars, faster than the corresponding increase in human care costs. (Smith 1994).[5]

Within the human health care sector, spending on nonprescription drugs, heating pads, bandages, and other items bought at retail outlets—products that do not require a prescription and are virtually never covered by insurance—rose 53 percent in real terms between 1980 and 1991: slower than overall national health spending, but almost twice as fast as GDP. Between 1960 and 1985, nonprescription-drug spending actually outpaced spending on prescription pharmaceuticals (and grew about 1 percentage point faster than real GDP; Letsch 1992).[6]

The seemingly inexorable rise in health costs has led to calls for a deliberate attempt to bridle cost growth. Although often couched in the rhetoric of efficiency savings, these proposals are intended to constrain health spending below the levels that would obtain even in an efficiently run health sector. Long-term cost containment proposals take the form of global budgets (as in the Clinton plan), expenditure limits (as in the American Health Security Act), or entitlement caps that only restrain spending in government programs, originally proposed by Richard Darman in the Bush administration (Marmor 1994). While their genesis is in very different outlooks on the health sector, they all respond to the same reality: health spending simply will not stop growing very rapidly because of *any* onetime efficiency-enhancing reform.

It is worth reiterating the four different types of evidence that support this point. First, as I discussed in the previous chapter, estimates of the potential savings from specific reforms suggest that they could not make substantial inroads into costs. Second, the roughly comparable rates of growth in other countries suggest that the peculiarities of the U.S. health sector do not explain the high rate of growth in costs. Third, the rate of growth in costs within the United States has been stable over a long period—six decades. Finally, spending in health-related areas such as veterinary medicine and nonprescription pharmaceuticals, where the peculiarities of the health sector loom less large, has also increased much faster than inflation. All of this evidence suggests that without external cost constraints, any attempt to improve efficiency in the U.S. system—whether a return to the high copayment rates that existed before insurance spread widely in the 1960s, a massive expansion in managed care, or an overwhelming reduction in administrative costs—will not make much difference in the rate of cost growth for more than a few years.

Reasons for Cost Growth: More and Better Technology

Health spending—in all of these sectors, in all of these countries, and throughout the twentieth century—has grown mainly because people want new and improved health services and the health care industry has been extraordinarily successful at satisfying that demand. Spending grows when new therapies with high dollar costs are initially developed. Spending also grows because of the diffusion of existing technologies. As physicians and manufacturers gain experience with new technologies, the unit costs of producing the technologies often fall, but the size of the population that could benefit from the technologies rises. The resulting increases in utilization often more than offset reductions in unit costs.[7]

In the 1980s, better treatment for early cancers spurred the use of sigmoidoscopies and breast biopsies (diagnostic procedures for colon and breast cancers) among Medicare patients. More convenient, less painful, quicker surgery encouraged the spread of outpatient knee surgery and lithotripsy for kidney stones (PROPAC 1993). From 1980 to 1990, as surgeons gained experience with coronary artery bypass techniques, the fraction of men over sixty-five undergoing heart bypass surgery in the United States quadrupled—from 1 in 400 hundred to 1 in 100 (CEA 1993).[8] Advances in fertility treatment sparked a threefold increase in the number of U.S. clinics providing in vitro fertilization services during the 1980s, although the nation's infertility rate remained constant and in vitro fertilization services are only infrequently covered by health insurance (DeWitt 1993).

Units of new technologies per capita are typically much higher in the United States than in countries with lower health care costs (Rublee 1989, 1994). Correspondingly, usage rates for these technologies in other countries are significantly below U.S. rates.[9] For example, in 1993 Canada had only about one-third as many open-heart-surgery units per capita as did the United States, and the rate of coronary artery surgery in Canada was one-third the U.S. rate (Rublee 1994; Azevedo 1993). Of the 51,500 implantable heart defibrillators (devices used in the treatment of some forms of heart disease) sold through 1992 in the United States, Japan, and Europe, 90 percent were implanted in the United States (Smith 1993).

One reason that technology usage in the United States is higher than in Canada is that the characteristics of patients on whom surgery is performed differ. In Canada, for example, fewer older patients (over age seventy-five), women, or patients with other complications have bypass surgery than in the United States (McGlynn et al. 1994). The greater use of costly technologies for elderly patients in the United States relative to other countries raises concerns that some of this additional use may be "wasted"—used in elderly patients who will die shortly with or without the costly medical intervention (McClellan, McNeil, and Newhouse 1994). But again empirical evidence does not support the view that such use is an important contributor either to the growth in U.S. health care costs or to the gap in health spending between the United States and other countries.

The share of Medicare spending on patients in their last six months of life held constant between 1976 and 1988, even as the level of spending on all patients exploded (Lubitz and Riley 1993). In other countries—even in Britain, where the government constrains resources especially tightly—the fraction of total health spending devoted to people over sixty-five is very similar to the comparable fraction in the United States (Heller, Hemming, and Kohnert 1986).

Furthermore, a growing body of evidence suggests that this higher rate of technology usage among the elderly does provide some benefits in terms of life expectancy. International statistics suggest that life expectancy at older ages, when high-technology medical interventions may be most effective, is strongly affected by higher health spending.

Indeed, life expectancy at age eighty in the United States ranks first among all countries (Bureau of the Census 1992).[10] By contrast, the United States performs very poorly in comparisons of life expectancy at birth and of infant mortality, measures that depend more heavily on social conditions and the use of routine medical treatments.

Moreover, many new and rapidly spreading health care technologies address primarily the quality of life, not its length. Hip replacement, knee replacement, cataract surgery, laparoscopic gall bladder surgery, and bypass surgery, among many other rapidly proliferating technologies, have much stronger effects on the quality of life than on life expectancy and are much more common in the United States than elsewhere (Azevedo 1993). Comparisons across countries suggest that in some instances the higher usage of costly interventions in the United States may contribute to especially good U.S. outcomes with respect to quality-of-life measures. For example, heart attack patients in Canada, who on average receive less aggressive treatment than their American counterparts, were 62 percent more likely than American patients to report experiencing chest pain and 55 percent more likely to report experiencing breathing difficulty (Mark et al. 1994). Patients who have had hip replacement surgery almost uniformly report that they are very satisfied with the surgery, but rates of the surgery are less than half as high in Canada as in the United States (Petrie, Chamberlain, and Azariah 1994; Azevedo 1993). Such technologies are costly, but they provide tangible benefits.

Measuring Health Care

The role of technology in improving the quality of life and reducing the suffering associated with medical procedures can help explain why technological change in medicine always seems to increase monetary costs. Many dimensions of health care costs are not reflected in the dollar costs alone. Similarly, an increase in the number of procedures performed, while fairly easily measured, is not an inherently meaningful indicator. A successful operation, involving little pain and a rapid recovery, should count for more than a painful, prolonged procedure that is only partially successful. Similarly, a drug that solves a problem without any surgery might represent a quality improvement over even the best surgery. Health care treatment, generally, is a fairly miserable part of life. In surveys monitoring the pleasantness of everyday activities, Americans rank it below doing laundry and homework (Robinson 1993). Quality improvements that reduce danger, pain, time demands, and other unpleasantness may have great dollar costs but they also result in substantial reductions in the nonmonetary costs of medicine. Yet only the dollars spent—not the nonmonetary savings—show up in cost accounts and spending-growth calculations.

A full accounting of the cost of health care should include these nonmonetary costs of medical practice (Newhouse 1993b). Consider time costs. Health care treatment consumes both patient time and the time of family and other voluntary caretakers. Patients spend time waiting for appointments, lying in bed in the hospital, and recovering at home from illnesses. The quality of their lives may be further diminished if that time is spent anticipating an uncomfortable or risky procedure or waiting for a diagnosis. Families spend time, including time taken from work, attending to sick members. None of these time costs show up in national health statistics.

Failure to account for the savings in patients' lost time and in family time can cause analysts to overstate the effect of many 1980s medical innovations on total costs. Outpatient surgery has reduced in-hospital time and allowed patients to recover and return to work more quickly. Increases in nursing home use provide another example of how accounting conventions lead to overestimates of the cost of health services. If a woman takes care of her own aged parent at home, the costs of her time are never counted. If instead she admits her elderly parent to a nursing home, the cost of care for the parent is added to national health expenditures (Fuchs 1986).

Another set of costs involve patient discomfort and pain. Although much of medicine remains painful, medical innovations have significantly reduced the discomfort and pain associated with many procedures and treatments. Medical-equipment manufacturers, like old-time dentists, compete by offering more comfortable devices for diagnosis and therapy (Smith 1993). The success of painless dentists suggests that most people are willing to pay for reductions in pain, yet savings in pain costs do not figure in the national health accounts.

In most industries improvements in productivity bring reductions in costs. Improvements in medical productivity also reduce costs, but typically these savings are not monetized. Instead, productivity translates into reductions in time spent in hospitals and in recovery, and in pain and discomfort. These cost savings may be substantial. The reductions in admissions and lengths of stay between 1982 and 1992 translated into a savings of 326,000 person-years not spent in hospital across the U.S. population in 1992, about 70 percent among patients under age sixty-five.[11]

While part of the value of time costs can be quantified using days saved, savings in pain, discomfort, and risk, which are more difficult to count, have been even more substantial. These reductions in nonmonetary costs, like reductions in dollar costs, lead to increases in the demand for medical services. People who would prefer to bear their symptoms if the alternative is a painful and risky procedure might willingly undergo safe, painless treatment. In this sense, the increases in demand for medical care that have occurred over the past 40 years can be readily explained by the traditional economics of supply and demand. The total price of medical care—including the cost in time, discomfort, and risk as well as money—has declined over this period, notwithstanding the enormous increase in money prices.

The nonmonetary costs of medical care become more important in driving the demand for health care when people face a smaller share of the monetary cost of procedures. In a market with pervasive insurance, consumers bear little of the monetary cost of treatment and providers compete by offering lower nonmonetary costs of service (Weisbrod 1991). Insurance protects patients from the financial price of medical care, but they continue to have to pay the nonfinancial costs (time, discomfort, and risk) themselves.[12]

The central importance of reductions in nonmonetary costs in recent increases in the demand for medical care is well illustrated by the case of a new gall bladder surgery, laparoscopic cholecystectomy. Conventional gall bladder surgery had a long, painful recovery period, including a three- to seven-day hospital stay, and left a one-and-a-half-inch scar. The new laparoscopic technique involves a short (one- to two-day) hospital stay, has a brief, nearly painless recovery period, and leaves no apparent scarring. The two procedures have virtually identical medical indications and complication rates.

An HMO in Pennsylvania examined its experience with gall bladder surgery in the three years after the development of the laparoscopic procedure (Legoretta et al. 1993). Although the laparoscopic procedure cost the HMO 25 percent less per patient, patients themselves paid nothing out-of-pocket for either procedure. Despite the per-patient savings through laparoscopy, the HMO saw its gall-bladder-related costs increase 11 percent over the three-year period. The incidence of gall bladder surgery had rocketed. Patients who had previously chosen to live with gall bladder disease (which often disappears by itself) when the alternative was a painful, prolonged procedure, now chose to have the operation. From a purely life-expectancy-oriented viewpoint, the increased number of procedures was unwarranted (Diehl 1993). From a financial standpoint, there was no change in the price facing patients and no change in demand should have been expected. Yet the decline in nonfinancial costs had immediate and significant effects on demand. Patients did not live longer but they experienced less pain and suffering.

The experience of increased use that came with the development of new, less painful surgical procedures in gall bladder surgery also occurred in other areas of medicine in the 1980s, especially in cataract surgery and treatment of kidney stones. In both of these areas, the most important components of the quality improvement were reduced discomfort and a shorter hospital stay, not an improvement in life expectancy (PROPAC 1993).

Saving Money through Regionalization and Inventories

The diffusion of technology brings complex equipment to Americans' hometowns and local hospitals. Almost 18 percent of all hospitals in the United States today have an MRI machine, more than twice as many as did in 1986, and more than one-quarter have a CT scanner (American Hospital Association 1994). In almost every area of the country, patients can undergo treatment in local facilities. By contrast, countries with more-centralized systems focus resources on facilities in a smaller number of places. Patients who may benefit from these costly technologies must then be transferred to the specialized facilities.

Centralizing technologies—known in the health services research literature as regionalizing—has two effects. First, studies suggest, patients who are initially hospitalized in facilities that do not provide a particular kind of service are generally less likely to receive that service than are patients initially hospitalized at the regional center (Blustein 1993; McClellan, McNeil, and Newhouse 1994). Thus, regionalization tends to reduce usage of particular services (although whether it reduces inappropriate use or simply reduces use altogether is harder to assess).

Second, regionalizing services increases the level of experience at the regional facilities providing those services. A considerable body of evidence suggests that physicians who specialize in performing one particular kind of service do a better job than those who perform this type of service only occasionally, either because the former learn with experience or because patients select the doctors with the most favorable experience (Donabedian 1984; Flood, Scott, and Ewy 1984; Leape et al. 1991). By encouraging patients to use experienced physicians, regionalization might improve the quality of service provision. Recent studies, however, suggest that this improvement is likely to be relatively small (McClellan, McNeil, and Newhouse 1994). Furthermore, any such improvement in quality comes at a cost. Patients must incur travel expenses and obtain care in an unfamiliar environment, often from doctors with whom they have no personal connection.

Patients frequently have the option of seeking care at a distant facility with providers who are more experienced than those nearby. Many do choose distant hospitals to obtain higher-quality care (Luft 1983; Phibbs et al. 1993).[13] Many others, though, choose not to do so, perhaps because they prefer to be cared for by physicians who know their personal history. In polls 57 percent of Americans report a willingness to pay more for local access to services (Jacobs, Shapiro, and Schulman 1993). While health planners agree that savings could be achieved by consolidating technology at regional centers, many Americans both speak and act as though they would pay more to have high-technology equipment available locally.

The spread of technology has also practically eliminated waiting time for most medical services. In other countries, delaying access to technology is a central element in the rationalization of resource use (Aaron and Schwartz 1984; Redelmeier and Fuchs 1993). Put simply, in the United States, equipment sits idle waiting for patients. In other countries, patients wait for equipment.

As in most industries, health planners must decide how to make the most effective use of costly capital equipment in the face of fluctuating demand for goods and services. In traditional manufacturing industries, the response to fluctuating demand has traditionally been the use of inventories. Plants attempt to operate at the highest possible level of their costly capital equipment's capacity and then store output (at some carrying cost) in anticipation of increases in demand. Clearly, this post-production, inventory-based approach does not work in a service industry like health care.

Using queues for medical services, though, is analogous to this process. Health planners assemble a preproduction "inventory" of service demanders and provide them with services at a rate that keeps all available capital equipment and resources (including highly trained physicians and other personnel) operating at maximum capacity. This system reduces the average cost of operating the capital equipment (because it is used so much), but imposes "carrying" costs on patients, who must wait for their turn. In other sectors, this method is like that used for charter flights that require ticket purchasers to buy nonrefundable tickets well in advance of flight time. The process ensures that flights will be full when they take off, but imposes costs (in the form of early commitment) on purchasers.

Potential savings in capital costs from using preproduction inventories are substantial. Capital costs in medicine take the form of training costs (human capital) and costs of physical capital. Once the costs of training physicians and purchasing equipment have been paid, the real cost of using these physicians and this equipment to produce one more procedure is relatively low. In the early 1980s, a CT scanning machine cost $700,000 to buy and $420,000 to staff and maintain each year, but beyond these expenses, it cost only $25 to perform one additional scan (Aaron and Schwartz, 1984). A scanner cost little more to buy and operate if it performed 500 procedures a week than if it performed only 50, and the hospital could recoup its fixed costs much faster in the former case. Savings achieved through more intensive usage of medical equipment and trained personnel may account for much of the lower cost of hospital care found when Canada is compared with the United States (Redelmeier and Fuchs 1993).

This preproduction inventory approach, however, is relatively uncommon in the service sector. In manufacturing, idle capital equipment is more costly to carry than inventory, but the opposite appears to be true in the service sector. The amount of fuel needed to fly the New York–Washington shuttle would be much lower if the shuttle simply waited on the ground until it had a full load of passengers. But passengers' waiting costs are high enough that they are quite willing to pay a substantial premium in exchange for knowing that the shuttle will depart at its scheduled time even if it is not full. A McDonald's franchise operates with far more burners and grill operators than would be needed if all food were prepared ahead of time and inventoried for future customers or if customers waited for their food to be prepared so that all burners and grill operators were in constant use.

There is no uniform answer to the question of whether patients' carrying costs are greater or smaller than the savings from more rational use of capital equipment. In other service sectors, two kinds of service are often observed. Some people's carrying costs are low enough that they would prefer to wait and purchase lower-priced services; in airline travel, these are advanced-purchase, economy-fare passengers. At the opposite extreme, others prefer to pay more and receive services immediately. In airline travel, these are business travelers, who pay the highest price in order to have the freedom to travel at short notice. Everyone recognizes that in the case of emergency procedures, patient carrying costs generally exceed savings from rationalizing capital use. Carrying costs for nonemergency procedures are likely to depend on the procedure and the individual.[14]

Waiting lines are often equated with central "rationing" of resources, and for most goods and services the existence of a waiting line does suggest that such nonprice rationing is being used. In most cases, nonprice rationing wastes resources by requiring humans to stand in line when resources could be more efficiently allocated using dollar bills. In health care, waiting lines have a more complex role. To the extent that they are used to generate preproduction inventories, they can reduce the average cost of health capital, even while raising patient costs in terms of time and inconvenience. Health care waiting lines represent a trade-off between patient costs and capital costs.

The trade-off of patient and capital carrying costs can be seen using estimates from a recent study on patient waiting times for knee replacement surgery in Canada and the United States (Coyte et al. 1994). The study found that waiting times from first seeking an orthopedic consultation to completion of surgery in Canada averaged 18.9 weeks—11.2 weeks, or 2.5 times, longer than the 7.7 weeks it took in the United States.[15] Some Canadian patients waited as long as one year for the surgery.

Costs of knee replacements in Canada were not provided in the study, but other estimates suggest that overall costs per hospital admission are about 30 percent lower in Canada than in the United States (Redelmeier and Fuchs 1993) and that a knee replacement in the United States on average costs about $12,000 (Healy and Finn 1994). This suggests that per-procedure knee replacement costs in Canada may be some $4,000 lower than in the United States. Canadians, then, trade off 11 weeks of serious knee problems (inability to climb stairs, for example) for $4,000 in savings, about $50 per day. Many individuals with a bad knee would gladly take this deal, but others would reject it, preferring to pay more to avoid the wait. In a system that rationalizes services by using queues, patients have no option but to accept the delay. If people have choices among health plans, those who place a lower value on delay can choose very restrictive health insurance plans that rationalize services using queues. Those who want services immediately can opt for more costly plans that provide services more quickly. For a number of conditions, Americans are much less willing than Canadians to wait a day to see a doctor (Blendon et al. 1995). More than three-quarters of Americans assert that they would not accept longer waiting times in exchange for lower health care prices (Jacobs, Shapiro, and Schulman 1993).

In general, Americans seem to place a high value on the benefits of technological innovation and the widespread availability of new services in health care. Survey evidence consistently shows strong support for expensive technology, conveniently and immediately available (Pauly et al. 1992; Ginzberg and Ostow 1994). Consumer choices in health care also vigorously endorse increased and immediate use of technology. One way consumers could voluntarily make trade-offs between costs and technology access would be by choosing HMOs that limit coverage for high-technology services. Instead, virtually all insurance contracts today offer access to the same technologies (Newhouse 1992b). HMOs can also ration access to technology through the use of waiting lines or regionalization.[16] In this light, it is interesting to note that the most rapidly growing managed-care arrangements, preferred-provider organizations and point-of-service plans, provide consumers with a safety hatch allowing them to obtain technology quickly even if their insurer does limit access.

While the adoption and diffusion of costly technology has occurred faster in the United States than elsewhere, a similar process occurs in other countries. The United States had a higher number of costly high-technology facilities per capita in 1987 than did either Canada or West Germany (Rublee 1989). All three countries, though, increased the number of these high-tech units in the early 1990s; in some cases, the rate of growth was faster in Canada and Germany than in the United States (see Figure 4.2). By 1993 per capita levels of many of these technologies in Canada and Germany were higher than the 1987 levels in the United States, although still below the 1992 U.S. per capita levels. While these countries may have postponed the cost of new technology for five years, they eventually incurred these costs as well. Despite their very different health systems, all three countries experienced continuing cost pressure as technologies were introduced and diffused.

Earlier adoption of technologies in the United States may mean that Americans waste money on procedures that turn out to be ineffective. It also means that the U.S. system improves the lives of some people who would not have had access to these technologies in other countries. The decision to adopt technologies early imposes costs—but so does the decision to wait and see.

Health Care Spending and American Well-Being

Advocates of cost containment might concede that the rising cost of health care can be explained by the adoption and diffusion of new technologies. But they might respond that rising health spending, however beneficial, hurts the remainder of the economy. The rising share of health spending in the GDP, after all, clearly limits Americans non-health spending. There is only 100 percent of GDP available to spend (aside from borrowing) and if the share of health care rises, something else must be falling. But the question is, what is falling and why?

Americans worry about a scenario in which the rising price of health care means that, on average, they must spend an ever-larger share of their income to buy the same treatment. But a rising share of consumption devoted to health care could be the outcome of many other processes. The quality of health care could be improving more rapidly than the quality of other goods, prompting consumers voluntarily to shift purchases away from other goods and toward health care. The prices of other important goods could be declining, leaving Americans with more income available to spend on health care and other discre-

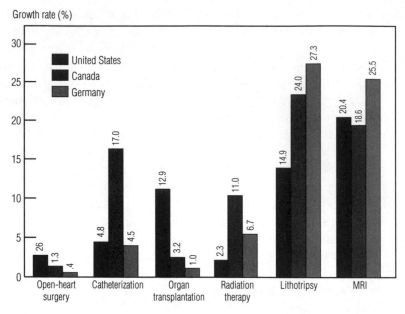

Figure 4.2 Recent growth in high-technology health care in three countries. Growth rates shown reflect the annual increase in the number of high-tech health facilities per capita. Data for Canada are for the years 1989 to 1993, except lithotripsy and MRIs, which are for the years 1988 to 1993. Data for Germany are for the years 1987 to 1993, except open-heart surgery and organ transplantation, which are for the years 1988 to 1993; for 1993 only, data include the former East Germany. Data for the United States are for the years 1987 to 1992. (*Source:* Rublee 1994.)

tionary purchases. Rising income could, by itself, shift consumption toward health care. In any of these alternative scenarios, rising health spending would be a sign of economic strength and well-being, not economic weakness.

An increase in the share of national income spent on health care represents a change in the composition of consumption (or savings), the basket of goods and services that people buy. The composition of consumption changes constantly, and health care is only one of many sectors whose share has increased steadily. Changing tastes, incomes, and prices have all contributed to the growth and decline of sectors.

The striking feature of U.S. spending over the past 50 years has been the rapid decline in the share of spending on food. In 1940 Americans spent almost 30 percent of their income on food. Today that figure has fallen by nearly half, to under 15 percent (CEA 1988, 1995). As Figure 4.3 shows, the decline in food spending from 1940 to 1990 completely offset increases in health care spending. But American consumers are not eating less food or lower-quality food than they once did. On the contrary, within the food sector the share of the less costly component, food eaten at home, has been declining while the share of the more costly component, restaurant meals, has risen. Americans spend less money on food because the relative price of food has declined. The combined figures for food and health expenditures show that Americans have been able to spend more on health care without drawing down spending on other goods. Instead, rising health spending simply offset the declining cost of food.[17] Of course, if health care costs had grown more slowly, the savings from lower food spending could have been spent on more automobiles or clothes or housing.

Even over the past decade, the aggregate consumption data suggest that rising health spending has not impaired the ability of Americans to purchase other nonnecessary goods and services. Between 1980 and

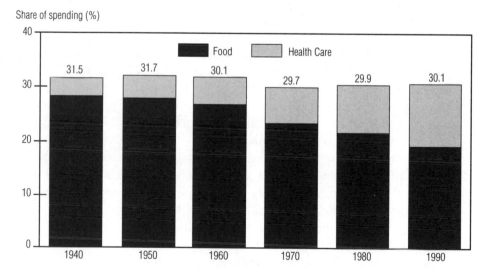

Figure 4.3 Food and health care spending in the United States as a share of personal-consumption expenditures 1940–1990. (*Source:* CEA 1988, 1995.)

1989, while real per capita health spending increased 47 percent, Americans bought 47 percent more jewelry, consumed 22 percent more restaurant meals, and spent 60 percent more on automobiles (McKenzie 1992). There is no evidence in the aggregate consumption data to suggest that rising health spending is crowding out other purchases. Again, if health care spending had not risen as quickly, Americans could have bought even more jewelry, restaurant meals, and automobiles. It is far from clear that such a shift, from replacement knees to replacement cars, would represent an improvement in national well-being. The evidence suggests that rising health spending has accompanied improvements in Americans' well-being and has not impoverished the nation.

These data represent the experience of the nation as a whole. Many families did find themselves putting off purchases of discretionary goods and services to pay for health care. But the problems that these families face are problems related to the distribution of health care expenses and income, not to the aggregate level of health spending. Large and increasing disparities of income among families in the 1980s and a lack of comprehensive insurance coverage meant that the experience of individual families diverged from that of the nation. The problems of individual families are quite distinct from the economic effect of a growing share of health care in national income.

While aggregate consumption data raise no red flags about rising health spending, many reform advocates have argued that the growing cost of health care has drawn down workers' paychecks, making it harder for them to buy the goods and services that they would like. Aggregate data show that as employers paid more of workers' total compensation in the form of health insurance, they paid less as wages and in other forms of fringe benefits (CEA 1993). Between 1975 and 1991, total real compensation per worker rose by 5 percent; but this sum masks an increase in average real wages per worker of only 1.3 percent and an increase in average real health benefit costs per worker of 132 percent (Cowan and McDonnell 1993). Advocates of cost containment note that if health care costs as a share of labor compensation had remained constant from 1975 to 1993, annual wages per employee would be $1,000 higher than they are today (CEA 1994).

Here, too, an awareness of growing disparities in earnings casts a different light on the statistics. Between 1980 and 1992, the real average hourly earnings of male full-time, full-year workers in the United States fell 0.3 percent; those of workers aged eighteen to twenty-nine with high-school educations fell 15 percent. Meanwhile, per capita health spending skyrocketed. Did this decline in wages represent a sacrifice of earnings for more costly health insurance? The answer, contrary to the standard rhetoric, is no. As Table 4.2 shows, male workers who were likely to have had employer-provided health insurance coverage in both 1980 and 1992 experienced virtually no decline in wages, and female workers in this group saw their real earnings increase nearly 9 percent. Male workers who never had employer-provided coverage, and whose wages should have been immune from the effects of rising health spending, saw their wages fall 1.8 percent. Those who lost insurance, and should have seen their wages rise accordingly, experienced an even larger 2.8 percent decline in wages.

Highly educated, experienced workers saw their earnings rise in the 1980s. They also received compensation packages containing more-

Table 4.2 Wages, health insurance, and wage growth for full-year, full-time U.S. workers, 1980–1992

Category	1980	1992	Percent change
Men			
Employer-provided insurance (%)	81	66	(15.0)
Average hourly wage	$14.40	$14.36	(0.3)
Average wage if insured in 1992[a]	$14.90	$14.87	(0.2)
Average wage if uninsured in 1980[a]	$12.99	$12.75	(1.8)
Average wage if insured in 1980 but uninsured in 1992[a]	$13.66	$13.28	(2.8)
Women			
Employer-provided insurance (%)	73	63	(10.0)
Average hourly wage	$ 9.82	$10.66	8.6
Average wage if insured in 1992[a]	$10.02	$10.93	9.0
Average wage if uninsured in 1980[a]	$ 9.25	$ 9.84	6.4
Average wage if insured in 1980 but uninsured in 1992[a]	$ 9.29	$ 9.86	6.1

Source: My computations, using data from the 1981 and 1993 Bureau of the Census Current Population Survey data tapes. Predicted employer-provided health insurance is computed based on education, age, age-squared, race, and region.

a. Predicted values are from multivariate analysis.

costly health insurance. During the same decade, the wages of workers with little education and experience declined substantially. Many in this group had never held employer-provided health insurance coverage. Others, facing the possibility of a further reduction in their wages, gave up their employer-provided coverage. Between 1980 and 1992, the fraction of male full-time workers receiving employer-provided coverage fell from 81 percent to 66 percent.

Rising costs of health care cannot be blamed for much of the decline in earnings experienced by workers in the 1980s. Rising health spending was concentrated among those whose earnings did not fall. Lowering the growth of health spending during the 1980s might have slowed the increase in the number of uninsured Americans, but it would not have increased the wages of less-educated American workers. Instead, it would have raised the amount of cash received by more highly educated, high-income Americans.

Health Spending and Productivity Gains

The data on consumption patterns over time highlight a possible explanation for the rapid increase in health costs without a contemporaneous decline in other kinds of consumption. The declining share of food in GDP is primarily a consequence of the falling price of food as the agricultural sector has become more productive over time. While in 1920 it took 90 person-hours to produce 100 bushels of wheat, by 1970 that much could be produced using only 9 person-hours (Department of Commerce 1975). Such improvement in productivity has driven down food prices. In real terms, food prices have grown much more slowly than wages. The average American worker can buy 53 percent more food from one hour's labor today than the corresponding worker could in 1940. Productivity increases in one sector, by reducing prices, may lead to increases in consumption in other sectors.

Productivity increases in some sectors may also lead to misleading estimates of increasing prices in others. The rise in health prices is partly a consequence of health care having become relatively more expensive as other goods and services have become relatively less costly. Because all prices are relative, when productivity in one industry improves, the relative price of goods produced by that industry falls and the relative price of goods produced by other industries rises.

Goods-producing industries have experienced much more rapid improvements in measured productivity than have service-producing industries. This effect of differential productivity growth across industries, first noted by William Baumol in 1967, means that the relative price of labor-intensive goods, such as Mozart string quartet performances, has risen dramatically over the two centuries—not because waste and inefficiency today characterize string quartet production, but because productivity growth has transformed agriculture.

Baumol cited medicine, along with education and city public services, as a sector where productivity growth would be relatively slow. He noted that the relative-productivity-growth phenomenon could lead to a situation where a growing fraction of the labor force would be employed in the production of low-productivity-growth services. The rising relative prices of medicine, education, and city services, along with the rising shares of employment in these sectors, are consistent with Baumol's hypothesis.

There is, however, evidence that tends to rebut the applicability of Baumol's hypothesis to medicine. Baumol would have predicted a widening gap between medical prices and other prices in periods of rapid productivity growth. Instead, exactly the opposite pattern occurred. Medical-care prices grew relatively more quickly in the 1980s, when economy-wide productivity growth was minimal, than they had in the 1960s, when productivity grew vigorously. Furthermore, the productivity of medical care has clearly improved, although most of these improvements (reductions in discomfort and time costs) do not show up in the medical-care price index—a shortcoming that renders the index rather meaningless (Newhouse 1993).

While Baumol's hypothesis explains little of the actual growth in health care prices in the postwar period, the basic point of his article is worth reiterating. The forces of productivity growth (combined with increases in the share of spending on health care as incomes rise) should be expected to push a greater share of income and employment into those sectors where productivity growth is relatively slow.

Competitiveness

Much of the concern about rising U.S. health costs centers on the effect of these costs on the nation's international competitiveness. Perhaps the United States can afford health care costs today, but if they continue to grow, advocates argue, American businesses will face an insurmountable competitive disadvantage relative to countries with lower health care costs. Executives in many large U.S. corporations have been quite vocal about how the cost of health care is making it difficult for them to compete overseas. Both President Clinton and Ira Magaziner, who ran Clinton's health care reform effort, found these statements quite compelling. Yet virtually all economists agree that in today's health system private health costs have no effect whatsoever on competitiveness (Reinhardt 1989).[18]

The argument that private costs do not affect the economy operates on two fronts. Health costs, in themselves, can affect competitiveness only if they lead to an increase in labor costs. In today's voluntary health insurance market, increases in health insurance costs almost certainly do not raise overall labor costs.

Firms may choose whether they wish to offer health insurance and how much insurance to offer. Similarly, workers have the option of working for a firm with or without this benefit. Firms are likely to offer health benefits only if they believe that their workers prefer these benefits to an equivalent increase in wages. If workers did not value health insurance at its full cost to employers, employers could attract more workers by offering somewhat higher wages and fewer health benefits.

The trade-off that workers make between health insurance and wages is readily apparent in union negotiations. Firms and unions today, looking back over a 60-year span of continually increasing health insurance costs, would be behaving extremely shortsightedly if they failed to make provisions for rising costs in their contracts. Instead, union leaders recognize the trade-offs between richer health benefits and higher wages. As early as 1960, industry-wide steel contracts explicitly noted that increases in health insurance costs through the duration of the contract would be taken out of the cost-of-living increases workers would otherwise receive (Somers and Somers 1961).

In a voluntary market, where workers bear the full (after-tax) cost of any benefits they receive, higher benefit costs will not affect total labor costs. More benefits simply mean a change in the composition of those labor costs, from wages to benefits. In turn, because labor costs do not change, the prices of a firm's products will be unaffected by increases in health insurance costs. If product prices do not change, then the ability of firms to sell their goods in other markets will also be unaffected.

Even if the argument sketched above fails, a backup argument based in international-trade theory suggests that any increases in health costs that did translate into higher labor costs would not affect U.S. competitiveness. Instead, any increase in the nation's average labor costs that is unrelated to productivity will translate into a decline in the value of the dollar. That decline in the value of the dollar will reduce the cost of U.S. traded goods to their original level. In this theory, an increase in health costs can affect the value of the dollar, but it cannot affect the ability of U.S. firms to sell their goods overseas.

The value of the U.S. dollar fluctuated dramatically during the 1980s. These changes, driven by differences in savings rates, speculation, and changes in trade balances, dwarf changes in relative health insurance costs over this period. Consider the experience of West Germany and the United States in the late 1980s. West Germany implemented numerous health reforms in the latter 1980s, bringing per capita costs down from 61 percent of U.S. costs in 1985 to 50 percent of U.S. costs in 1990, an 18 percent drop. Meanwhile, though, the exchange rate fell from 2.94 to 1.62 deutsch marks per dollar, increasing relative German export costs by more than 50 percent. In an environment of rapidly fluctuating exchange rates, it seems very unlikely that small, gradual changes in relative health care spending would have any measurable effect on American competitiveness.

The theoretical arguments above are consistent with a wealth of empirical evidence. Within the United States, total labor costs as a share of national income have remained steady over time, despite the escalating cost of health insurance (see Figure 4.4). Increased spending on health insurance has displaced growth in other components of workers' earnings. Put differently, workers have purchased more health insurance over time. Rather than purchasing it after receiving their wages, they have had it deducted from their paychecks before receiving their pay in dollars. Rising health insurance costs are borne by workers who have health insurance, not by U.S. businesses.

The evidence from within the United States is bolstered by data, compiled by the U.S. Bureau of Labor Statistics, that compare labor costs in 30 developed countries. These hourly labor costs include wages, insurance and other benefits, and payroll taxes. Comparisons

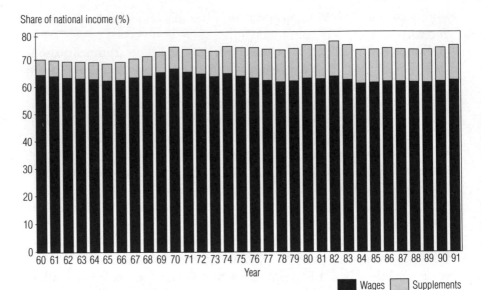

Share of national income (%)

Figure 4.4 Wages and wage supplements in the United States as a share of national income, 1960–1991. (*Source:* CEA 1994.)

among countries are made using average exchange rates over the year. Despite much higher per capita costs for health insurance, U.S. relative labor costs consistently rank well down among these countries (Department of Labor 1991b). More compelling still, despite rapidly rising health insurance costs in the U.S. manufacturing sector during the 1980s, labor costs in the United States *fell* relative to these other countries.

Complaints about the effects of rising health costs have come most persistently from the automobile industry (Iacocca 1988). Executives of the Chrysler corporation complain that health care costs them over $700 per car, $300 to $500 more than their overseas competitors (Maher 1990). Ford Motor executives note that health costs per car are much lower in Canada (Graig 1993). A number of economists have sympathized with these concerns, on the grounds that highly unionized industries, such as auto manufacturing, may have more difficulty transferring rising costs to workers (Aaron 1991; Thurow 1984).

A simple examination of the effects of rising health spending on competitiveness comes from looking across the border. In the Canadian provinces, health insurance costs are paid through taxes that do not depend on the actual health costs of a particular worker or firm. The terms of the 1965 U.S.–Canada auto pact require U.S. automobile firms to produce at least 75 percent as many cars in Canada as they sell in Canada. As a consequence, all three U.S. automobile manufacturers have large automobile plants in southwestern Ontario, across the border from Detroit. If health insurance costs are an important contributor to the lackluster export performance of U.S. cars, their Canadian subsidiaries should be booming, and facing far less import competition. Car companies should endeavor to move their production facilities, to the extent possible, across the border to Canada.

This has not happened. Instead, unions in Canada negotiate for higher wages while union negotiators in the United States negotiate for more generous benefits. In the United States in 1991, 37.3 percent of labor costs went to pay benefits, while in Canada, only 26.7 percent went to benefits. Average pre-tax hourly labor costs, including both wages and benefits, were almost the same on both sides of the border, and Canadian costs had been rising relative to U.S. costs. Canadian manufacturers have been equally vulnerable to overseas competition. The share of non–North American–produced cars among all cars sold was slightly higher in Canada in 1988 than in the United States (Motor Vehicle Manufacturers' Association 1992). As Figure 4.5 shows, production of passenger cars in Canada has fluctuated as a share of the North American market; but it has not done so in any manner consistent with rising relative health expenses in the United States.

Business leaders have complained most vociferously about the cost of employee health insurance policies that provide benefits to retired workers. Before they retired, these workers accepted lower wages (or made other concessions) in return for the promise of these benefits in the future. Many firms may have miscalculated in offering these benefits, believing that growth in health costs would slow. The concessions that they wrested when they promised the benefits may have been too small.

To put it another way, firms made an investment when they offered retiree benefits to their workers. They took a loan from their workers that they promised to pay off at a variable interest rate determined by

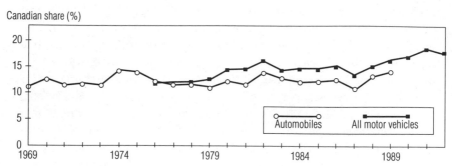

Canadian share (%)

Figure 4.5   Canadian share of U.S.–Canada motor vehicle production 1969–1992.
Source: Ward's 1990; Motor Vehicle Manufacturers' Association 1992.

the future cost of health care. Had they correctly estimated the cost of care, or, better still, overestimated the costs, their investment would have been a profitable one. The interest rate they signed up for would have turned out to be equal to or lower than the market rate. Unfortunately for American business, many took a loan with a fluctuating interest rate that wound up higher than they had anticipated.

Current workers did not sign the contracts providing benefits to previously retired workers. Just as it would be unlikely for current workers to make significant wage concessions because their firm took a loan at an excessively high interest rate, there is no reason to believe that current workers would be willing to accept lower wages so that their employers can continue to pay the cost of these policies.

Similarly, customers of the firm's products are unlikely to accept higher prices to compensate the firm for its errors, whether those errors are called retiree health benefits or high-interest-rate loans. Instead, the cost of these errors generally falls on the shareholders of fumbling firms.

The cost of retiree benefits represents a loss to shareholders of firms offering these benefits. Losses to shareholders do not affect international competitiveness, just investor pocketbooks. When the government offers to reduce these costs by shifting the burden to taxpayers or by spreading it among all firms, it enriches shareholders at the expense of everyone else.

The potential gain to shareholders of firms with outstanding retiree-health-benefit liabilities are substantial. A federal accounting-rule change effective in 1993 required firms to list the amounts of their liabilities on their balance sheets. Overall, these figures amounted to $402 billion in 1988, including future liabilities for current workers. Not surprisingly, investors appear to take these liabilities into account when making their purchase and sale decisions. Analyses suggest that the share value of companies falls about 50 cents for every dollar they owe in retiree health obligations (Mittelstaedt and Warshawsky 1993).

The Federal Budget Deficit

The need, real or perceived, to trim the federal budget deficit motivates much of the concern over rising health costs. The federal Medicaid program spends more money on poor Americans than all other federal poverty support programs (Aids to Families with Dependent Children, food stamps, Supplemental Security Income, housing vouchers) combined. One in every three dollars paid to elderly Americans by the federal government arrives in the form of medical care through the Medicare program (OMB 1994). Over the 1980s, both the federal Medicare and Medicaid programs grew at annual nominal rates of over 11 percent, considerably faster than the federal budget or the economy as a whole. Today, Medicare costs make up 11 percent of federal spending, while Medicaid spending accounts for a further 5.8 percent (CBO 1994a). Political liberals whose agendas stretch beyond health care are disheartened by the fact that existing health program obligations stymie their ability to spend on other, potentially more productive initiatives (Brown 1993). Fiscal conservatives observe that the tax reductions they favor are impossible, under balanced budgets, without health cost containment.

Both groups look to cuts in government health programs to address their concerns. Unfortunately for their mutual cause, there is little evidence that increasing profligacy accounts for the rising cost of either of the major government health programs.

In the 1980s, the Health Care Financing Agency (HCFA), the arm of the Department of Health and Human Services that operates the Medicare program, implemented significant institutional innovations aimed at cost containment on both the hospital and physician side of medical spending. In 1983 HCFA implemented the DRG payment system, paying hospitals according to a patient's diagnosis on admission, independent of the particular services provided by the hospital. The DRG payment system gave hospitals powerful incentives to limit the services they provided patients. In 1992 HCFA began using a payment system for physicians that increased the fees paid for evaluation and management procedures and decreased those paid for interventions. The new payment system also contained a mechanism to adjust for increases in the volume of procedures. If the volume of procedures performed in one year exceeds the level projected by HCFA, the fee scale is automatically reduced in the following year to maintain total payments at the expected level.

These institutional payment innovations have made it possible for Medicare to achieve substantial savings from fee reductions. Hospitals and physicians now find it more difficult to repackage procedures and increase the volume of services rendered to keep payments up when fees are reduced. Such fee reductions have been an important feature of federal health policy throughout the 1980s and 1990s. Between 1985 and 1992, the per-diagnosis fees Medicare paid to hospitals rose more slowly than the CPI every year (PROPAC 1993). Congress froze physician fees between 1984 and 1986. Similar programs to reduce costs are now envisioned for other provider payments in Medicare.

Prospects for additional forms of institutional savings in the Medicare program are slim. Administrative costs in the program are very low, less than 1.4 percent of claims in the hospital insurance program, even lower than those in the Canadian single-payer system (Etheridge 1992; Social Security Administration 1992). Experience with the use of HMOs in Medicare suggests that, at present, only limited savings can be achieved by moving more Medicare beneficiaries into HMOs (Brown et al. 1993).

Overall, payments per Medicare beneficiary rose slightly faster than per capita health expenditures in the early 1980s and slightly slower after cost containment began in earnest in the later 1980s. Medicare cuts in the 1993 budget imposed further substantial fee reductions over the remainder of the decade. Whatever the merits of these fee cuts from a health policy perspective, from a budget perspective they will yield only a 1.5-percentage-point decline in the rate of growth of Medicare. Increasing use of costly procedures means that, despite budget cuts, program costs per beneficiary will continue to grow about 3 percentage points faster than per capita GDP.

Funding for the Medicaid program is split between the federal government and the states, who administer the program. Mandated coverage expansions, providing coverage for poor children and pregnant women, as well as the recession and decline in employer-provided coverage, meant that the number of Medicaid beneficiaries increased 22 percent between 1989 and 1991 (Letsch et al. 1992).

States took a number of steps to reduce their cost of the Medicaid program. Medicaid payment rates are already very low, about 50 percent of private rates (Physician Payment Review Commission 1995). To further reduce costs, some states enrolled nonelderly beneficiaries in HMOs. By 1992 about 15 percent of Medicaid beneficiaries belonged to HMOs. States also increasingly used a range of accounting tricks to shift the Medicaid burden more heavily onto the federal government, a development that makes it difficult to assess the contribution of other factors to rising per capita Medicaid costs (Letsch et al. 1992). Nonetheless, the evidence suggests that despite the states' varied efforts to suppress Medicaid cost growth, costs per beneficiary in the program rose almost as rapidly as private health care costs during the 1980s.[19]

The recent experiences of the Medicare and Medicaid programs suggest that cost containment, whether achieved by blunt measures such as drastic Medicare fee cuts or through incentive-based approaches like encouraging enrollment in HMOs, cannot halt the advancing front of higher spending in these programs. Unfortunately, the structure of financing for these programs means that funding will always lag behind spending.

General revenues fund the federal contribution to Medicaid. Increases in the cost of medical care, even without changes in coverage, mean that Medicaid draws more and more from the federal funding pool. In addition, the coverage expansions of the 1980s were not explicitly financed. No tax was raised and no specific program cut to pay for Medicaid expansions. Instead, Medicaid expansion meant that the program drew a larger share of the government's general revenue pool.

The Medicare program is financed in a more complex way. The Medicare trust fund, which collects taxes from employers and employees, funds Medicare hospital spending. Employer and employee premium rates have increased steadily over the length of the program, from 0.5 percent each in 1967 to 1.45 percent each today (Social Security Administration 1993). Despite its characterization as a "trust fund," the Medicare fund does not, in general, save premiums to pay for future health costs. Rather, current premium income defrays current health spending. When health care costs rise, Congress must increase taxes accordingly.

General revenues and premium payments from Medicare beneficiaries fund the Medicare supplementary insurance program. Between 1967 and 1993, the federal government's need for general revenues to fund the Medicare supplemental program and Medicaid program increased by a factor of 20 as a share of GDP; from 0.1 percent of U.S. GDP to almost 2 percent of GDP (OMB 1994).

Medicare premium payments for medical benefits originally paid for 50 percent of the cost of these benefits. Over time, however, the premiums were increased only by general inflation while costs grew at the rate of medical inflation. By 1983 Medicare Part B premiums paid for only 25 percent of the cost of Part B benefits. Since 1982 premiums have been frozen at 25 percent of the cost of benefits. Had Medicare beneficiaries paid 50 percent of Part B costs in 1993, Medicare's draw on general revenues would have been $13.5 billion lower, a difference that accounts for 5.3 percent of the 1993 budget deficit.[20]

The relationship between federal health spending and the budget deficit occurs not because government health costs in general are unusually high (compared with private costs) or because federal health program managers are particularly ineffective or spendthrift, but because the financing of these programs has not kept pace with their expenditures. The types of financing used for health programs grow along with general tax revenues. Health care costs, in both the public and private sectors, however, grow much more quickly than these revenues, producing a ballooning gap. Since this pattern is familiar in other countries as well, analysts assert that general-revenue funding of health programs consistently leads to increases in both health spending and government deficits.[21] Given the political reluctance to saddle people with additional taxes or to cut benefits in existing programs, general-revenue financing for health care, regardless of the health system chosen, is a prescription for growing budget deficits (Hoffmeyer and McCarthy 1994).

If Costs Don't Matter, Why Do People Complain?

The empirical evidence suggests that Americans have been spending more on health care and getting more services—services that they seem to value highly—in return. Rising health care costs cannot be fairly blamed for a decline in American living standards, a weakening of the competitiveness of the U.S. economy, or growing budget deficits. Nonetheless, policy analysts of all stripes point to cost containment as central to the health debate. Furthermore, Americans, when surveyed, always complain about the cost of health care (Jacobs, Shapiro, and Schulman 1993). Can the enormous difference between perceptions and realities be reconciled?

It is worth noting that people have been concerned about the high cost of health care since the first poll was conducted in 1937 (*Gallup* 1937). If actions are evidence of intentions, concerns over health costs date back at least to the time of Hammurabi, who fixed the fees doctors could charge ("Survey" 1991). In 1983, when health care consumed 10.5 percent of the GDP, 65 percent of Americans complained that health care costs were too high, and virtually the same percentage complained in an identical poll eight years later, when costs had risen to above 13 percent of the GDP. As Herman and Anne Somers noted in 1961: "It is often pointed out to the disgruntled consumer that while he is paying more, he is getting a better buy for his money than ever before; he is receiving a better quality of medical care and more of it. This has not proved sufficient assuagement. Even if he appreciates the fact that he is receiving a far better product, it does not necessarily make it easier to pay for" (p. 217).

Americans tend to respond in much the same way in other sectors where costs are rising rapidly. In periods when overall inflation is high (the only time pollsters ask the question), a majority almost always favor wage and price controls (*Gallup*). When oil prices rose rapidly in the 1970s, a surprising number of Americans polled supported gas rationing.[22]

Given a choice between current prices and lower prices, holding everything else the same, any rational person would prefer lower prices. At the same time, when asked to make trade-offs between higher prices and the amenities of a health service (such as waiting times, more technology, or local technology), most people appear to prefer to spend more in exchange for getting more. Health insurers have the option of selling plans that limit purchasers to 1970s technologies but charge only 1970s prices. They do not do so, presumably because few people would choose this option. While Americans may complain about rising health care costs, they also insist that the nation should be spending more, not less, on health care (Blendon et al. 1995).

Concern about overall health spending may simply disguise other policy goals. People may favor reductions in costs if they expect that the level of spending will remain the same but the incidence will be redistributed away from them. Business interest in reducing obligations for retirees falls into this category. Shareholders do not care much about cost containment generally, but they would prefer to transfer the retiree obligations they bear to taxpayers generally.

Public-policy makers gain on two fronts from cost containment strategies. First, in an atmosphere where taxpayers believe cost containment can be achieved without sacrifice, restraining health costs is a politically popular way of getting money to spend on other programs. Second, rigid cost containment strategies make it easier for reformers to predict the costs of the plans they propose and hence their effects on the federal budget. Experience with implemented health programs, including Medicare and Medicaid, which exceeded their budgeted costs very soon after they began, has made lawmakers quite reasonably wary of passing open-ended, unfunded legislation. But this emphasis on producing programs with predictable cost implications has dangers. Heavily regulated programs with severely controlled costs have more predictable budgetary implications than do less regulated programs. An emphasis on predictability might make policymakers more willing to adopt a heavily regulated program even when a less regulated program would be preferable.

Cost containment may also advance other political agendas. Conservatives like the idea of a budget limit on public health expenditures because cutting such entitlement spending reduces the size of government. Many liberals believe that a global budget, especially a comprehensive one, could reduce inequities in the system by constraining spending at the top end. For example, in the name of controlling spending under a national budget, the Clinton plan included limitations and prohibitions on billing above government-established medical fee schedules (a practice known as balance-billing). By thus restricting the amount that the rich could possibly spend out-of-pocket on medical care, these limits would presumably reduce disparities in access between rich and poor.

Global Caps

Caps on national health spending have been incorporated in a number of reform proposals (see CBO 1993b for a discussion of some of these proposals). In President Clinton's health plan, spending for all services included in the national benefit package was to be constrained by a budget limitation (technically, a cap on premiums). By limiting spending on an expansive range of services, the plan could ensure that national health spending in the United States would slow as a share of GDP. As in most plans, the global budget would not only cover most health spending but would also include rigid and automatic provisions to ensure that spending remained within preset limits.

At first, mandated spending limits in a global budget could probably be met by eliminating services that people do not value very highly. But if an enforceable global budget were implemented, it would eventually constrain spending by indiscriminately slowing the introduction and diffusion of costly new health technologies, regardless of their value. The potentially absurd implications of such an outcome confirm the notion that a rising share of health spending in GDP does not represent a problem and should not be controlled.

Imagine, for example, that a cure for breast cancer were found that cost $25,000 more per case than current treatment methods. Full implementation of the cure would increase the share of health spending in GDP and violate a global-budget restriction, but it seems very unlikely that society would be better off delaying implementation.

An advocate of automatic limits in global budgets might argue that in such an eventuality, politicians could choose to relax the budget prohibition or reduce spending on some less efficacious medical treatment. Imagine, then, a technology that enabled all childhood vaccinations to be given orally, at an additional cost of $5 for each of the six sets of vaccinations a child receives before age two. The technology would not improve (or diminish) health outcomes, it would not increase the number of children vaccinated, and it would not increase anyone's productive work time, but it would save children some of the misery that today accompanies vaccinations and it would increase the share of health care in GDP by a tiny fraction (0.002 percentage points). Given a choice, most parents would probably be willing to pay the extra $30, even if it meant reducing their child's consumption of candies or toys.

Technologies that cost more but reduce discomfort are constantly being developed and would, eventually, violate a global-budget limitation. Where a particularly costly technology yields substantial benefits, the political process might relax the budget rules to accommodate the technology. But the steady flow of minor improvements in the comfort or ease of care, valued by some consumers and largely ignored by most, is unlikely to lead to revisions of the budget. The very existence of the budget, in turn, is likely to stymie the development of such desirable technologies.

Careful evaluation of new and existing technologies, increased provider and patient sensitivity to costs, and reductions in inappropriate use of technologies would reduce health costs and increase health benefits. Cost containment strategies advocated by both medicalists and marketists that pursue these goals are laudable. But eventually, any strategy that vows to keep costs as a share of GDP under some fixed ceiling simply for the sake of cost containment will require sacrifices in the form of worse health outcomes, higher time costs, or more pain and suffering.

Before such cost containment proposals are accepted, a case has to be made that, as a society, Americans cannot afford to spend more on health care. No evidence available today supports that case, and forecasts for the next 40 years show no signs that this situation will change. Analysts currently predict that health care spending will rise to 32 percent of the U.S. GDP by the year 2030 (Burner, Waldo, and McKusick 1992). Even so, the projections suggest that real per capita GDP exclusive of health care will also continue to grow, at a rate of 0.8 percent per year. If the projections are correct, Americans will be buying more health care, but they will also be buying more of other valued goods and services.[23]

Until now, the rising cost of health care has been associated with an increase, not a decline, in the well-being of most Americans, because it reflects improvements in the quality of care. Furthermore, national health expenditures have no effect on the competitiveness of the U.S. economy. All the evidence points one way: if Americans choose to do so, they can, as a nation, afford to spend more on health care.

5 ///

How Much to Whom?

Much of the debate about health reform has centered on improving the efficiency of the health system and reducing total health costs. But the prospects for achieving substantial savings through improving efficiency are slim and policies that use brute force to constrain spending are likely to make people worse off. The principal effects of any health reform are not likely to be on how much Americans as a nation spend on health care. Rather, they will mainly affect who pays for that spending and who receives its benefits. Such redistributional issues get less press than proposals for saving money. Redistributing resources is less politically palatable than promising to improve efficiency and make everyone better off. Yet fundamental aspects of most health reform proposals—insuring the uninsured, community rating health insurance, and financing the Medicare program—all call for substantial redistributions of resources.

Redistribution in the health care system takes three forms: redistribution between the healthy and the sick, redistribution within the middle class by age or region, and redistribution from high-income to low-income Americans. Each of these types of redistribution has grown in importance as the costs of medical care have risen and as the organization of health financing and delivery has evolved.

As late as 1966, before the great expansion of public health insurance coverage, most Americans paid their health expenses out of personal savings or by borrowing and repaying money.[1] Poor people received some care funded by charity, but for the most part, little redistribution took place through the health system. In the postwar period, this self-insurance system began to be replaced by private health insurance that pooled the costs of health spending among a larger group of people. Private health insurance began to transfer money from the healthy to the sick. State- and federally funded medical-care programs, financed through broad-based taxes, made redistribution through the health system more explicit. Today, most people's health payments bear little relationship to their current use of health services.

The Healthy and the Sick

In any given year, most people use very few health services. The 1 percent of Americans with the highest spending on health care in 1987 accounted for fully 30 percent of total health spending in that year. By contrast, the 50 percent of Americans with the least spending accounted for only 3 percent of total health spending (Berk and Monheit 1992). In fact, about 15 percent of Americans use no health care in any given year (Lefkowitz and Monheit 1991).

This pattern is not a consequence of any particular feature of the U.S. health system. Researchers find similarly concentrated spending in France and Canada (Aaron 1991). While the concentration of spending has increased somewhat over time, even in 1963 the 50 percent of Americans with the lowest health spending accounted for only 5 percent of costs (Berk and Monheit 1992).

What has changed is the dollar amount of health spending and the relationship between spending on health and average incomes. The 1 percent of Americans with the highest health spending in 1963 spent an average of $11,000 each on health care, only about 10 percent more than average disposable personal income in that year.[2] By 1987 the most costly 1 percent of American medical-care consumers spent an average of $63,000 each on health care, more than 3.5 times average personal income in 1987. The rising cost of health care, combined with the underlying skewedness of health costs, suggests that Americans are unlikely to return to a time when health care is financed primarily through personal savings.

The financing of health spending is considerably less concentrated than the use of health services. Most people's health insurance premium payments, out-of-pocket expenditures, and health-related taxes fall within a narrow range. While out-of-pocket expenditures are more concentrated than premium or tax payments, they have not become markedly more concentrated over time. In both 1977 and 1987, about 10 percent of the U.S. population spent more than 10 percent of their income on medical care, and in both years, most of this group had low incomes (Taylor and Banthin 1993).

Redistribution and Private Insurance

If health spending were completely unpredictable, a health insurance system would transfer funds paid by people who turn out to be healthy to those who turn out to be sick. While such a system would transfer funds, it would not require explicit political decisions about how much healthy people should contribute to the care of those who are sick. When people bought health insurance, they would do so without knowing how much health care they would need. On average, they could expect their health care premium to equal their health care spending.

But health care spending is not completely unpredictable. High health spending tends to persist over time. Having certain health conditions today raises the risk of having high health spending in the future. Many people who have a serious illness one year do have few health expenses in later years, so, over time, health spending evens out a little. But it remains quite lopsided (Zook, Moore, and Zeckhauser 1981). Over a 1-year period, the top 1 percent of Medicare spenders account for 20.3 percent of spending; over a 16-year period, the top 1 percent (in that sixteen year period) account for 7.2 percent of spending (Gornick, McMillan, and Lubitz 1993). Lifetime health costs are higher for those who are born with or develop a serious illness or disability than for those who do not.

Spreading the costs of those with easily predicted higher health spending to those with lower spending expectations goes beyond the kinds of transfers that can occur naturally in a purely private health insurance system. Healthy people will not voluntarily choose to buy health insurance coverage that costs much more than their expected health expenditures. If people who expect to have high costs are to be

covered at affordable rates, the healthy must be persuaded to contribute
to the care of those who can be expected to be ill.

Health Security

The issue of "health security," which received a lot of attention in the
1993 health reform debate, implicitly addressed this question of redistribution between the healthy and sick. Middle-class Americans with
good health coverage expressed a concern that if they became ill they
might be unable to obtain health insurance coverage at reasonable rates
(Newport and Leopard 1991). In a recent survey, 25 percent of Americans polled responded that someone in their household failed to
change jobs because of a fear of losing health coverage (CEA 1993).

Many analysts have argued that health insecurity has been increasing
as the insurance sector has changed. They assert that when most insurance premiums were community rated, offering the same rates to
everyone regardless of health status, the problem of health security did
not exist. Over the past two decades, though, most plans that had community-rated their insurance policies (primarily Blue Cross plans) have
switched to experience rating, where insurers adjust premiums to cover
the costs expected to be incurred by a group. The premiums needed
to cover some illnesses may be so high that they effectively close off a
portion of the market. This pattern was exacerbated by the passage of
federal legislation in 1974 (the Employee Retirement Income Security
Act, or ERISA) that, in effect, encouraged firms to self-insure the health
coverage that they provided to their employees. Under self-insurance,
employers (rather than insurance companies) make all the payments for
their employees' health expenditures—a form of 100 percent experience rating.[3]

Many of those in ill health who do obtain coverage find that their
insurance fails to cover their health conditions. Health insurers today
typically exclude from coverage (at least for some period) conditions
that preexist the health insurance contract. In 1994 more than 60 percent of conventional insurance contracts included such preexisting condition clauses (Gabel et al. 1994). Furthermore, some self-insured companies also refuse to hire or insure people with preexisting conditions
(OTA 1991).[4] Those in very bad health may be unable to obtain health
coverage at all. Hillary Clinton's reaction to this situation sums it up

well: the way insurance works, "only the healthy would be insured" (Clymer 1993).

The actual extent of the health security problem is difficult to gauge. Some empirical evidence does suggest that those in poor health have to pay a relatively higher surcharge for insurance coverage now than they did in the late 1970s.[5] But studies also find that few uninsured people have ever investigated the cost of coverage. In 1987 only 37 percent of the uninsured had investigated coverage; only 2.5 percent of the uninsured were ever denied coverage or offered only limited coverage because of a health condition (Beauregard 1991).[6]

The Origins of Risk Rating

The growth of experience rating undoubtedly made life more difficult and costly for those in ill health who sought insurance, but the problem has a long history. Critics who complain that the rise in the number of uninsured in the 1980s "can be largely laid at the door of the private insurance companies risk-management strategies" (Ginzberg and Ostow 1994, p. 84) echo their counterparts in the early 1960s, long before the expansion of self-insurance. In 1961 writers lamented "the triumph of experience rating," which made it impossible for "millions" at high risk to purchase insurance coverage (Somers and Somers 1961, p. 406). Experience rating and preexisting-condition clauses are not a modern aberration; they are a natural and integral feature of a competitive, voluntary health insurance market.

Insurers behave in ways that mean that those who are in poor health pay more for health coverage (or obtain less coverage at a given price) than do healthy people. Risk-based selling and pricing of this form is not unique to health insurance markets. Homeowners in earthquake zones cannot buy home insurance from private insurance companies; people who are terminally ill cannot buy life insurance; and drivers with very bad records cannot buy automobile insurance. Indeed, incentives for risk-based selection exist whenever heterogeneous consumers pay providers a standard flat fee for services rendered (Newhouse 1992a). Hospitals prefer healthier patients under a DRG system: they cost less and bring in the same fee. Rent-regulated landlords prefer renters without pets or children: they pay the same rent but do less damage to apartments. Risk-based screening does not reveal the venality of the insurance industry; it allows insurers to survive.

Insurers price their policies according to the average payment they expect to make to policyholders. Policyholders who expect to receive a higher-than-average payout find it most valuable to purchase coverage. Homeowners in earthquake zones are much more likely to want to buy insurance coverage at average prices than homeowners in areas without earthquakes. As insurers cover more and more high-risk people, the average expected payout, and thus the premium, rises. Eventually, people who do not expect to be hit by earthquakes will stop buying policies. Only those who live on fault lines will have (very expensive) home insurance. The fact that high-risk people are more likely to buy insurance at average prices than are low-risk people is known as adverse selection. Adverse selection raises the prices paid by high-risk people and reduces the amount of insurance coverage purchased by low-risk people.

Risk-based pricing and selling changes this dynamic. By determining the characteristics of their risk pool, insurers can sell more generous policies to low-risk people at a sufficiently low price to make them willing buyers. To keep low-risk people in the pool, they offer them better prices than those offered to high-risk people. That leaves high-risk people with coverage at costs that reflects their full risk, but the price may be so high that they decide not to purchase coverage at all.

Both adverse selection and its consequence in the health market, risk-based pricing, stem from the fact that people have information about themselves that they can use in purchasing health insurance contracts. Once this kind of information exists, it becomes impossible to maintain a pooled insurance policy that offers all holders the same coverage at the same premiums in a competitive environment with voluntary purchase.

Many people's immediate response to the problem of risk-based pricing and selling is to require that insurers charge the same premiums to everyone they cover: a return to community rating. Virtually every health reform plan contains provisions designed to at least limit risk-based pricing in health insurance markets, through rate bands and limitations on preexisting conditions. While these plans may reduce the spread of rates between those at high risk and those at low risk in the same plan, they cannot eliminate the effects of selection. As long as people can choose to opt out of the market altogether, some low-risk people will avoid buying coverage at average prices and prices will be forced up. If insurers cannot respond to differences in risk that are known to those who buy insurance, individuals will. Adverse selection can cause the insurance market to disappear altogether as only those at highest risk purchase insurance.

This extreme outcome rarely occurs in actual insurance markets. Although private information exists in health care, most illnesses and accidents cannot be fully anticipated. Concern about the financial risk of illness is enough to persuade most people who have assets worth protecting that they would be wise to buy health insurance coverage. Most low-risk people do choose to pay average prices for extensive insurance. Adverse selection in the health insurance market, by itself, is unlikely to leave most people uninsured (Pauly 1985).

The structure of today's insurance market also reduces adverse selection. Most people today obtain coverage through employment-based group policies, which typically include people with different health statuses. The prices of these policies are based on the average cost for those enrolled. While the prices of employment-based policies change if a group member becomes sick (a serious problem in small firms), coverage within groups is more or less community rated.

If people can choose among many community-rated or rate-band-limited insurance plans, though, adverse selection may again undo the effects of employer groups, mandated community rating, or rate band regulations. This could lead to an outcome in which those at higher risk are charged substantially higher rates for insurance. High-risk people will prefer generous coverage, but low-risk people will often choose to buy policies with very high deductibles or significant restrictions on use, in part to avoid being grouped with those at high risk. Eventually, the price of the more generous insurance plans will increase, reflecting the more costly average experience of those enrolled in these plans. Evidence from programs that offer multiple insurance choices suggests that this kind of selection may occur. High-risk people in multiple-choice plans buy more generous coverage and pay higher rates than do those at lower risk.[7]

Why Risk-Based Pricing Is a Problem

In economic theory, risk-based pricing and selling is preferable to adverse selection. While high-risk people pay higher prices in either event, under risk selection low-risk people do buy comprehensive coverage, while under adverse selection they do not. Risk-based pricing allows everyone to buy insurance at actuarially fair prices. Much of the concern about health insecurity stems from a sense that while risk-based pricing may be actuarially fair, it is plain vanilla unfair. While those who drive poorly or choose to live in earthquake zones can adjust their behavior to avoid risk, the risk of developing many serious health conditions cannot be fully avoided. Risk-based pricing may be appropriate in the auto insurance or home insurance markets, where risk depends on the actions of the insured, but not in the general health insurance market.

This commonsense feeling has a formal analog. In today's health insurance market, even under risk-based pricing, low-risk people cannot buy truly comprehensive insurance: insurance that covers the risk of future illnesses. People who are healthy today cannot buy a policy that will lock in their future insurance premiums even if they develop a health risk later.

Solutions to the Risk-Selection Problem

Risk selection can be eliminated if everyone is required to participate in the same insurance pool and buy identical policies, as happens in countries where basic insurance coverage is provided to everyone or is compulsory. While there may be problems of risk selection in the market for supplementary coverage in these settings (where such coverage is permitted), being sick does not affect the cost of basic health coverage in these systems.

Avoiding risk selection is more complicated in a private, competitive, noncompulsory insurance system. To date, there have been only limited private and regulatory efforts to address the problem. To some extent employees do lock in their health insurance through their employers when they are young, and as long as they remain with the same employer, they are protected from future increases associated with new health conditions. But employees who change jobs lack this kind of protection in the employment-based U.S. health insurance system. Recent legislature changes (the Health Care Availability and Affordability Act of 1996) help ensure that job changers have access to health insurance but do not protect them against premium increases. In the life insurance market, people avoid problems of risk selection by buying lifetime coverage when they are young—before they know how healthy they will be later. The option of buying when young does not work as well in the health insurance market. Insurers have not developed lifetime health insurance or multiyear fixed-premium products for individual purchasers. In part, the tax subsidy for employer-provided insurance has limited the market for long-term individual coverage. Most middle-class people, even those who currently purchase individual coverage or are uninsured, expect to be employed by a firm that offers health insurance at some point, and this reduces their interest in purchasing long-term private insurance today.

A long-term health insurance policy might promise to pay policyholders who develop a covered condition a fixed annual amount. The amount per condition would reflect the surcharge that an average insurance company would charge to cover a person with that condition (with some copayment). For example, if the average insurance company charged people who had ever been diagnosed with skin cancer $1,000 extra a year for coverage, the long-term policy might pay policyholders diagnosed with that disease $800. Policies would be sold primary to young people who had not yet developed any adverse health conditions. Like life insurance contracts, these policies would require individuals to make higher payments at young ages and commit themselves to paying premiums that would later increase only with the average rate of health costs. Such long-term contracts could ameliorate many of the problems associated with adverse selection and risk selection in health insurance, as they do in the life insurance market.[8]

Long-term contract purchases could reduce health insecurity without requiring explicit transfers from those who know they are healthy to those who know they are sick. But long-term purchasing would not work for everyone. For example, it would not work for those whose health conditions are already evident when they are young—a group, which while relatively small today, may grow as genetic testing improves.

Absent long-term insurance contracts, efforts to reduce the high rates paid by those in ill health, whether because of risk selection or adverse selection, do require explicit transfers from the healthy to the sick.[9] Explicit transfer policies constitute forms of risk adjustment, or regulatory redistribution, between the healthy and the sick. Risk adjustment is a system of payments between health insurance plans intended to adjust for differences in the risk of those enrolled in different plans. Plans that enroll mainly healthy people make payments to those that enroll a higher proportion of people with serious health conditions. In principle, under such systems insurers do not care whether they enroll mainly sick people or mainly healthy people. Healthy people cost them less in medical payments, but require them to make more payments into the risk pool, while sick people bring a reward in the form of transfers from the risk pool.

Risk adjustment creates a dilemma. Sharing the expense associated with high-cost cases among insurance companies reduces each insurer's incentive to select healthy policyholders, but it also reduces each insurer's incentive to monitor the cost of care. For example, full-risk adjustment, whereby all plans share equally in the cost of all cases, completely eliminates the incentive to select by risk, but it also eliminates each plan's incentives to keep costs down. Incomplete-risk adjustment leaves higher-risk people paying higher premiums. No one has ever designed an ideal method of risk adjustment, one with a risk adjuster that would optimally balance cost containment incentives and risk spreading. Furthermore, risk adjusters, even imperfect ones, have not been used extensively and would be technically complex to establish and monitor.

The existing health insurance market has not resolved the problem of redistribution between the healthy and the sick. The extremely skewed distribution of ill health in the population means that the problem will persist under almost any health reform. Even a single-payer program without HMOs or competing conventional insurers would eventually require a system of risk adjusters if providers were paid on a capitated basis, by diagnosis, or through annual budgets. Otherwise, providers could offer longer visits, more pleasant service, and shorter waits at the same price if they recruited mainly healthy patients.[10]

In the absence of market solutions, such as long-term health insurance contracts, which might address the problem of risk-sorting in health insurance without government intervention, explicit decisions must be made about redistributing resources to the sick. All redistributive transfer programs, whether pure community rating, rate bands, or risk adjustment, have inherent technical deficiencies. Forcing insurers to set prices without regard to risk can encourage individuals to sort themselves according to risk, so that sick people pay higher rates. Spreading risk widely may diminish incentives for cost containment. But besides the technical problems of designing redistributional mechanisms, regulatory solutions force people to confront the question of which transfers from healthy to sick are appropriate.

How Much Redistribution to the Sick?

Medicalists, who emphasize the role of the medical system in determining health, would argue that fairness requires equal payments without regard to risk. Marketists, who emphasize the role of the individual in generating health, argue that people should be responsible for at least some of their own health outcomes. The threshold of this debate today is whether health insurance premiums for cigarette smokers should be the same as those for nonsmokers.[11] Prior to recent court rulings, some businesses, using similar reasoning, dropped coverage for HIV-related illnesses from their health insurance packages. Some employers today penalize employees who are overweight or fail to control their blood pressure (Bernstein and Garland 1990).

These problems will only grow as more is learned about health and medical care. The range of potentially avoidable health outcomes is already quite long and will lengthen as medical science improves its ability to predict the health consequences of behavior. In turn, the existing consensus in favor of reforms that spread costs from the healthy to the sick may weaken. Failure to reform risk-based pricing could improve the nation's physical health: while future medical costs may figure only marginally in the decision to pursue a risky behavior today, an immediate increase in health insurance premiums might be effective in deterring risky behavior. Smokers may not worry about the costs of lung cancer when they decide to smoke, but an increase in health insurance premiums today, like a tax on smoking, is likely to affect their decisions. At the same time, though, genetic testing and other diagnostic techniques mean that people are likely to know more about their health status in the future than they do today. That would make the problems of adverse selection or risk-based pricing worse and further diminish health security.

Redistribution within the Middle Class

From the Young to the Old

My discussion of redistribution from the healthy to the sick focused primarily on unanticipated illness. But the most significant kind of redistribution from the healthy to the sick in today's health system, and in many proposals for reform, involves redistribution in the context of easily anticipatable illness. Almost everyone is healthy when they are young and almost everyone uses medical care when they are old. People over sixty-five spend, on average, seven times as much on health care as do those under nineteen, and about three times as much as the average American does (Waldo et al. 1989).

The high rates of use among the elderly are not related to the eccentricities of U.S. health financing. In France health spending for people over sixty-five is more than three times the average (Heller, Hemming, and Kohnert 1986). Even in Britain, where age is an explicit consideration in the allocation of some health resources (Aaron and Schwartz 1984), spending by those over sixty-five swamps spending by younger people by a factor of more than three to one (Heller, Hemming, and Kohnert 1986).

Relative health care costs among the elderly have increased slightly over time in the United States, in part because of the expansion of insurance coverage to people over sixty-five. In 1958 those over sixty-five spent about 1.9 times as much as the average American on health expenditures (Somers and Somers 1961). People over sixty-five, however, had much more difficulty purchasing insurance than other Americans. Those over sixty-five with health insurance in 1958 used about 2.4 times as much medical care as the average person. By 1977 the Medicare population over sixty-five used, on average, about 2.8 times as much medical care as the average American.[12]

While the elderly account for over 35 percent of U.S. personal health spending, they pay far less than one-third of all health bills.[13] Forty-five percent of the expenditures of people over sixty-five are paid by the federal Medicare program. Almost two-thirds of the funding of the Medicare program comes from payroll taxes paid by working Americans, more than one-quarter comes from general revenues (broad-based taxes), and less than one-tenth consists of payments by the elderly.[14] The Medicaid program, funded through general revenues, pays for an additional 12 percent of elderly health spending. Supplemental private insurance, along with out-of-pocket expenditures, accounts for the remaining 43 percent of spending.[15]

This funding pattern means that patterns of health care utilization and of health care spending diverge considerably. Under today's health insurance system, average private health insurance premium payments for people under sixty-five increase with age (Department of Labor 1986). Payroll contributions to Medicare rise with income but end at retirement. Thus, while health care payments, including Medicare premiums and the employer share of individual health insurance premiums, peak among older working people, health care utilization continues to increase throughout retirement (Waldo et al. 1989). As Table 5.1 shows, the average U.S. household headed by a twenty-five- to thirty-four-year-old pays more for health care than does the average household headed by someone over sixty-five.

The rising cost of health care, combined with the changing size of birth cohorts and differences in life expectancy, means that this financing scheme generates significant redistributions of income. The 20.5 million working uninsured Americans pay Medicare payroll taxes that cover health insurance for their elders, but the 0.5 million American households over sixty-five with incomes above $75,000 a year pay only the flat Medicare Part B premium (Department of Commerce 1993; EBRI 1993). While today's elderly did pay into the Medicare system when they were working, those payments do not come close to financing their current health expenditures. For a sixty-five-year-old man who earned average wages throughout his life, Medicare can be expected to pay out four times as much in lifetime Part A payments as the value of all payments he and his employers made into the trust fund, including interest on earlier contributions (House Ways and Means 1993). Even for those who made the maximum contributions to the trust fund throughout their lives, Medicare lifetime spending exceeds the value of contributions by a factor of about two.[16]

Workers today pay much higher Medicare payroll taxes than their elders did. In 1967 employers and employees each paid 0.5 percent of earnings up to a cap into the Medicare trust fund. By 1986 the em-

Table 5.1 Components of health spending for young and old households in the United States

Type of spending	Amount spent annually	
	25–34 years old[a]	Over 65 years old[a]
Out-of-pocket expenditures, including Medicare Part B premiums for those over 65	$1,030[b]	$2,257
Employer payments for health insurance	$1,491[c]	0
Tax subsidy for health insurance purchase	($447)[d]	0
Medicare payroll tax payments	$895[e]	0
Total	$2,969	$2,257

a. Age of head of household.

b. Of this figure, $317 is the out-of-pocket share of health insurance premiums.

c. For people aged 25–34, the average premium payment for an employer-sponsored plan was $2,750 (1987 figure updated to 1991 using the CPI and rate of growth in health spending). Employers paid 84.6 percent of the premium for this coverage (Cooper and Johnson 1993). In 1991, 68 percent of those 25–34 had private health insurance, of which 6.7 percent was privately purchased (EBRI 1993).

d. Employer payments multiplied by 0.30 to adjust for tax subsidy.

e. Median money income for families headed by people aged 25–34 was $30,845. Medicare taxes were 2.9 percent of wage-and-salary income.

ployer and employee rates had nearly trebled, to 1.45 percent of pay each. Since 1986 Congress has paid for spending increases by raising the earnings cap, and in 1993 it repealed the cap altogether. Today, high-income earners and their employers together pay 2.9 percent of all earnings into the Medicare system. Marketists argue that these high taxes have deleterious effects on the functioning of the U.S. labor market.

The Medicare financing system, which pays for the health expenses of today's elderly through a tax on today's young, also implicitly taxes future generations, who will have to pay for the future health costs of today's workers (Auerbach, Gokhale, and Kotlikoff 1993). The magnitude of these cross-generational transfers depends on the relative sizes of each generation, the rate of increase in health care costs, and continuing willingness to support the system. The cost of funding the elderly has relatively little impact on today's young people, because there are 4.8 working-age adults for every person over sixty-five (CBO 1993a). By 2030, when the last of the baby boomers has passed sixty-five, there will be only 2.8 working-age adults to pay the health costs of each person over sixty-five.[17] Their burden will be even greater if the aging of the baby boomers speeds the development of even more costly health care technology.

Many health reform proposals incorporate further intergenerational transfers. An expansion of Medicare for the elderly, either through provision of long-term care or pharmaceutical coverage, based on the existing financing scheme, would increase payments by the current and future young to the current and future elderly. Similarly, community rating health insurance, without adjustments for age, would redistribute income from those in their twenties and thirties to those in their forties and fifties.

Proponents of the current Medicare funding system, including medicalists (and many economists), point to the family ties that bind older and younger Americans to argue that these redistributions are irrelevant. Children may wish to provide their parents with good things. Parents can compensate their children for high future taxes by leaving bigger bequests. Governments, though, cannot write enforceable contracts that bind future generations. Many of today's baby-bust generation doubt that the Medicare program, in its current form, will be there to fund their health expenses when they get old. If they are right, they will pay twice for health care—for the care of their parents and for their own care.

Dismantling a redistributive financing system later on means leaving those who depended on its existence in a fragile position, without either savings or private coverage. Yet today, while the baby boomers are still in their prime earning years, Americans are already beginning to observe forays into the universality of social programs for the elderly. High-income earners can expect to get back only 25 cents of every dollar they paid into the social security system (House Ways and Means 1992). Proposals to tax or limit Medicare benefits for middle- and high-income taxpayers are already under consideration (CBO 1994c). Baby busters may be right to question the permanence of the Medicare program.

Redistribution among States

The second source of redistribution among the middle class implicit in any national health program is redistribution of health resources among the states. Health services and health needs differ dramatically across the United States. Maryland has almost three times as many doctors per capita as does Idaho; Massachusetts has more than twice as many dentists per capita as Mississippi; North Dakota has three times as many hospital beds per capita as Alaska. Infant mortality is 90 percent higher in Mississippi than in Massachusetts, and New York had 1,404 times as many AIDS cases per capita as North Dakota in 1993 (DHHS 1993). These differences in needs and resources, along with other area-specific factors, translate into substantial differences in health spending. In 1982, for example, Massachusetts spent 75 percent more per capita on health care than did Idaho (DHHS 1988). Even within the Medicare program today, spending per beneficiary in Alabama exceeds that in nearby South Carolina by more than one-third (PROPAC 1993). Differences in per capita health spending are a recurring theme in the debate about a new formula for allocating federal Medicaid funds.

The logic of "national" health reform suggests that Americans should spread resources more evenly across the population of the entire country. Variations in health resources, though, may reflect historical differences in the way states have chosen to allocate money. Public policy can ignore these preexisting allocations, in which case disparities in health resources will be perpetuated indefinitely, always leaving those states that began with few resources behind. Alternatively, policy can try to even out regional differences, which may mean overriding local preferences about the allocation of resources (Roberts and Clyde 1993).

Regional variations in utilization occur, in part, because of practice-pattern variations (as I described in Chapter 3) and historical differences in health resources. But quite a bit of the variation in service utilization arises because of the geography and culture of communities themselves. About one-third of regional differences can be explained by the density of the population: the time costs of seeking medical care significantly reduce use in rural areas (Welch 1992). Regional variation also reflects differences in attitudes toward health and medical care. States vary substantially in other health-related behaviors. The traffic fatality rate in Arkansas is 2.4 times as high as that in Connecticut; 32 percent of West

Virginia residents smoke, but only 15 percent of Vermonters do (Department of Transportation 1991; Van Son 1993).

A national health insurance scheme would obscure cross-state behavioral differences. Under a national financing system, rural residents who rarely seek care pay higher taxes to fund expenditures in states with patterns of more aggressive care-seeking behavior. Residents of states with high utilization rates must reduce them to national averages, even if they would prefer to pay more and maintain their traditional high use patterns.

From the Rich to the Poor

Redistribution from the healthy to the sick, from the young to the old, or from one state to another takes place mainly among members of the middle class. From a political perspective, this focus on redistribution within the middle class is understandable, but from a health policy perspective it makes little sense. The most significant health policy question in the U.S. health care system is how to provide care for low-income people.

In 1993, 37 million Americans, more than 16 percent of the population under sixty-five, reported that they had no health insurance (CEA 1994). Most uninsured people have low incomes. Fully 60 percent of the uninsured have low family incomes, below $30,000 (200 percent of the poverty mark) for a family of four; 90 percent have gross individual income below $20,000 (EBRI 1993). A slim majority of the uninsured are members of families that include a full-time worker (in part because many of the very poor, single mothers qualify for Medicaid). Uninsured workers, though, earn very low pay; in 1991, 81 percent earned less than $10 an hour (in 1989 dollars; Levit, Olin, and Letsch 1992).

In 1980 fewer than 30 million Americans, 13.7 percent of the population, lacked insurance coverage. During the 1980s, the rate of uninsurance among full-time workers increased by 28 percent. The rate of uninsurance among dependents of full-time workers rose even faster. This increase, however, occurred almost exclusively among workers earning relatively low wages. In particular, there was no increase at all during the 1980s in the rate of uninsurance among those earning $15 an hour or more (in 1989 dollars). Both in 1980 and in 1991, that rate stood at 2.9 percent. By contrast, uninsurance rates rose very quickly among those earning $6 an hour or less. In 1980 this group constituted 42 percent of the working uninsured. In 1991 it made up 52 percent of the latter group (Levit, Olin, and Letsch 1992).[18]

It is critical to recognize the centrality of low income—as opposed to systemic failures in the health insurance market—in the problem of the uninsured. If the problem of the uninsured were mainly a consequence of insurer risk selection or adverse selection, it could be remedied by tinkering with the health insurance market. It is not. Consider the recent experience of young Americans. While the rate of uninsurance in the population as a whole increased 16 percent during the 1980s, this group experienced very large increases in uninsurance. Among those people aged nineteen to twenty-five, the fraction uninsured increased by 25 percent, while for those aged twenty-five to thirty-four the fraction uninsured increased by more than 50 percent. In 1991, 47 percent of the uninsured were aged nineteen to thirty-four (Levit, Olin, and Letsch 1992).

The decline of community rating in the 1980s, along with the increased use of experience rating, self-insured plans, and preexisting-condition clauses during the decade, should have led to an increase in the relative propensity of young people, who are mainly healthy, to obtain health insurance. Young people's relative premiums would have *declined* as costs became more closely related to underlying health risk. Instead, young people stopped purchasing insurance coverage simply because their incomes fell. The average real hourly wages of male full-time workers aged eighteen to twenty-nine fell 14 percent between 1980 and 1992 (my computations, based on data in Department of Commerce, *Current Population Survey*).

Most people who do not have health insurance can not afford to buy the standard insurance package at market prices. That was true in 1957 and in 1976 and it is, if anything, more true today. Figure 5.1 compares the rates of uninsurance relative to family incomes in 1957, 1976, and 1991. The data have been adjusted to remove the effect of economy-wide inflation. Large declines in uninsurance among the lowest-income families occurred between 1957 and 1976, when public programs grew. The relationship between family income and insurance status among middle- and upper-income families became stronger between 1957 and 1976 and again between 1976 and 1991.

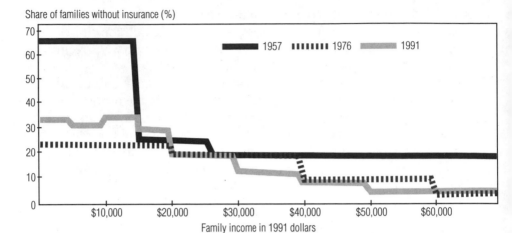

Figure 5.1   U.S. family income and levels of uninsurance in 1957, 1976, and 1991. All income figures have been converted to 1991 dollars using the CPI. Data for 1976 and 1991 do not include the elderly, who comprised 9 percent of the population in 1957. Adjusting for the elderly, 67 percent of whom were uninsured in 1957, would have little effect on the trends shown. (*Sources:* Data for 1957 are from Follmann 1963; data for 1976 are from CBO 1979; data for 1991 are from EBRI 1992.)

In 1957, as today, low-income families without health insurance did not go without health services. The U.S. health care system has always incorporated a de facto safety net for those who do not have insurance. Physicians and hospitals provided more than $25 billion in uncompensated care to uninsured patients in 1991, an average of $700 per uninsured person.[19] Between 1980 and 1991, hospital uncompensated-care payments grew at an annual rate 37 percent faster than total hospital spending (CBO 1993c).

Overall, Americans without health insurance use about 60 percent as much health services as do those with health insurance (after one controls for their demographic characteristics; OTA 1994). That differential means that providing the uninsured with the average insurance package would have increased national health spending by about $45 billion.[20] If that cost were spread across the entire population of the United States, the average American family of four would have to pay almost $600 more a year in taxes.

Of course, that $45 billion figure assumes that society provides the uninsured with the equivalent of what those who pay for their own coverage currently purchase. Providing the poor with less care would cost less. The basic question in extending coverage is defining what should be provided.

Who Gets How Much?

American policymakers have tried hard to avoid politically volatile questions about how much health care to provide to beneficiaries of public programs. Medicare, Medicaid, and many reform proposals limit payments to doctors and hospitals rather than explicitly restricting quantities of services. This strategy permits policymakers to fall back on calls for efficiency and ignore the question of limiting services. But all health plans must, at least implicitly, define the scope and range of constraints on the entitlement they offer, if only for budgeting purposes. The continuing growth in health care costs means that the $45 billion bill for covering the uninsured this year will escalate in the future. The need to address cost growth means that every health reform plan contains provisions somewhere that spell out who will be subject to limits on spending.

Every health care system—public or private—places restrictions on the entitlements it provides. In today's nonuniversal system, neither privately insured nor uninsured Americans have an open-ended call on health resources. Insurance policies include coinsurance or deductibles, many policies contain lifetime limits on service use, and managed policies monitor the use of other services. The uninsured may not be able to buy private health care at all. For privately insured and uninsured Americans today, rationing occurs through the price system. But a reform that promises universal coverage simply cannot leave all rationing decisions to the price system. Someone outside the price system must determine what "universal" coverage covers. That person or institution rations services centrally.

In some countries, such as Canada, central rationing (administered by the Canadian provinces) governs the availability of health services to virtually all Canadians. Regulations strongly inhibit the operation of a private market, so everyone is subject to the same limits. Other countries, including Great Britain and Germany, who use a weaker form of central rationing, only limit services paid through the public entitlement and permit residents to purchase private insurance and health services. In a two-tier system of this type, not everyone gets the same care.[21]

Countries with national health systems control the size of the entitlement both by directly restricting the quantity of health resources available and by restraining pay to health professionals as a means of indirectly limiting the services offered. In the United States, both the Medicare and Medicaid programs have used fee controls almost exclusively as a means of containing the size of the entitlement. Neither program directly controls the quantity of health resources available, and rules limiting the availability of particular services have only rarely been used in U.S. public programs.

Medicalists and marketists differ sharply in their views of central rationing. The rationing principles that appear in the health plans they propose are grounded in their very different views of what health care is.

Medicalists and Redistribution

To medicalists, need for care alone should determine use. Since individuals have only limited control over the state of their health and their need for health services, every person should be entitled to as much health care as is necessary, regardless of his or her income or other characteristics. Here, the medicalist view fits quite closely with popular sentiment. In opinion polls almost all Americans agree that everyone should have equal access to the best possible health care (Jacobs, Shapiro, and Schulman 1993, citing a 1990 poll).

As I suggested in chapter 2, it is not at all clear that needs alone determine health care use. Variations in treatment patterns suggest that patient preferences and physician training have substantial effects on the care a patient receives. The variations literature directly complicates the entitlement question: Should an entitlement to care reflect the treatment recommendations of a bold, high-cost physician or those of an equally qualified conservative, low-cost physician?

The nonmechanical relationship of treatments to conditions suggests that use of health care services will differ among people even in a fully insured market according to choice of physician, patient preferences about their health, and patient attitudes toward risk. Moving away from a strict identity between needs and use, many medicalists acknowledge these variations but reject variations according to income.

Nonmedical Interventions

As the benefits of health care shift from prolonging life toward improving the quality of life, trade-offs between the costs of medical and nonmedical responses become more acute. Throughout medical history, physicians have recommended that patients rest, travel, move to mountainous or dry climates, eat special diets, or avoid certain foods. In Germany national health insurance covers a biannual two-week spa vacation (GAO 1993b). Massage has been shown to benefit premature infants (White-Traut and Goldman 1988). Asthmatics benefit from dust-free housing (Call et al. 1992). These quasi-medical responses may be more effective in improving health than medical ones.

In many instances, nonmedical goods and services may even have stronger effects on life expectancy than differences in access to medical services. According to tests conducted by the U.S. Department of Transportation, the likelihood of a head injury in a 35-mile-per-hour crash is more than 6 times as high if you are the driver of a Chevrolet Lumina four-door sedan equipped with seat belts than if you are the driver of a costlier four-door Audi 100 with an air bag (Department of Transportation 1991). The standardized mortality rate for homicide in central Harlem, an area of high poverty, is 14 times as high as the national average (McCord and Freeman 1990). For middle-aged men, smoking cigarettes (which is twice as popular among those with incomes under $10,000 than those with incomes over $50,000) more than doubles the probability of dying within the next 16.5 years (Viscus, 1994).

Moreover, there is no substantial evidence suggesting that equality of access to medical care generates equality of health outcomes. Evidence from both Great Britain and Canada suggests that the gap in health outcomes between rich and poor adults has not substantially narrowed and in some instances has actually widened in the period since the introduction of national health insurance (Manga and Weller 1980; Goldblatt 1989; Wilkins, Adams, and Brancker 1989).

The disjunctions between medical needs, nonmonetary costs, and subjective benefits of treatment raise questions even where medical treatment would be medically beneficial. The value of a cataract operation is greater for someone whose passion is reading as opposed to listening to music. Arthroscopic knee surgery benefits athletes more than couch potatoes. Members of religious groups that shun medical treatment receive no benefits from a health care entitlement. Extremely poor patients may experience a greater improvement in their quality of life from adequate housing or even free movie tickets than from aggressive health treatment. By treating health care as special, medicalists would subsidize people who seek medical interventions for their problems, in a society that does not provide comparable assistance to people who prefer nonmedical treatment for similar problems.

For many years, the Sunday magazine of the *New York Times* has periodically included an advertisement that solicits readers who have trouble climbing stairs. The product advertised, a kind of mini-elevator, helps those with knee problems ride up the steps of their homes or offices. Today, knee replacement surgery can solve many of the problems that used to make people have trouble with stairs, albeit at greater cost. In effect, knee replacement surgery transforms the mini-elevator into an implantable device.

Few, if any, medicalists argue that everyone with knee problems should be entitled to a mini-elevator, and the machine's manufacturer was targeting a high-income market when it chose to advertise in the *New York Times Magazine*. According to the medicalist model, though, the transformation of this product from an external device to an internal one changes its status—from an ordinary consumer good into a form of health care—and means that it should be made available to anyone who would gain significant health benefits from it (or to no one at all).[22] Yet some poor people might prefer the mini-elevator to an implanted knee, and many would prefer the elevator if it were cheaper and they could keep the price difference.

Health Care and Other Public Benefits

In an era of tight public coffers, the decision to treat health care as special may result in denying funds to other programs that needy people might prefer. Proponents of an egalitarian approach to health resource allocation often recognize that more money for health care may mean less money for other programs. Many value health spending more highly than other spending or believe that health program beneficiaries will make shortsighted or inappropriate choices with nonhealth benefits. Health egalitarians appear willing to accept the trade-off of more health care and less of other goods and services.

One illustration of this medicalist view emerged from a theoretical discussion in the context of President Clinton's health proposal. In a system of multiple competing plans with different prices, poor Americans would have to be given a subsidy to buy coverage. Medicalists argued that the poor should be allowed to choose any plan they wanted, regardless of cost. This position would mean that, in many cases, the poor would be in plans that were more expensive than people who were not subsidized. As deficit hawks pointed out, the subsidy would be very expensive.

Falling back from this position, medicalists suggested that each plan be required to enroll a fixed fraction of subsidized people. On average, poor people would receive average benefits, but this would be accomplished by placing some in high-cost plans and others in low-cost plans. The coveted spots in high-cost plans would have to be allocated by lottery or some other nonprice mechanism among the population of those with subsidies. Lotteries, while they would break the income taboo, might create a situation in which some subsidy recipients "won" places in high-cost plans in locations that they found inconvenient. Furthermore, those whose incomes increased beyond the subsidy range might have to switch down, choosing less costly plans than those they had previously been entitled to through the lottery.

Alternatively, medicalists suggested subsidizing the poor up to the cost of the average plan in each area. Managed-competition advocates disliked this scheme because it gave the poor, unlike the nonpoor, little incentive to choose low-cost plans. Troublemakers proposed that those with subsidies simply be given a rebate if they chose a cheaper-than-average plan. This, of course, pleased neither public health advocates nor deficit hawks. Medicalists recognized that if the poor were given a rebate for choosing a lower-cost plan, most would choose the lower-cost plan and use the cash to buy other goods and services. Although this would have been an outcome generated entirely by the choices of those receiving subsidies, medicalists found it unacceptable. Politicians and deficit hawks feared that taxpayers who might be willing to pay for a health care subsidy would find a health care rebate uncomfortably close to direct income redistribution.

Pragmatic Egalitarians

While medicalists believe that strict equality is desirable for its own sake, many also favor a broad scope of rationing for pragmatic reasons. By requiring that all higher-income Americans receive the same care as the poorest, they expect to preserve the quality of care in the program.

Pragmatic egalitarians sometimes use a comparison of Medicaid and Medicare to illustrate this point. The Medicare program, which provides coverage to both the poorest and the richest Americans sixty-five and over is safeguarded by a powerful and vocal lobby of upper- and middle-income seniors. Medicaid, which covers only the poor, depends on the kindness and compassion of members of Congress, not their self-interest. Medicare beneficiaries can see the physician of their choice, while Medicaid pays such low rates to physicians in many states that beneficiaries have no access to private physician care at all.

A careful examination of the experience of the past 20 years, though, provides less support for the argument that universality helps the poor. Unlike the social security program, which provides income to people to spend as they wish, Medicare and Medicaid entitlements depend on the characteristics of the benefit package. The Medicare benefit package has remained virtually unchanged since passage of the legislation that created it, despite significant changes in private contracts. It contains substantial coinsurance and deductible provisions and does not cover pharmaceuticals. Middle- and higher-income elderly Americans buy supplemental Medigap coverage to protect themselves from these expenses. Lower-income elderly Americans who do not qualify for Medicaid face substantial and rising out-of-pocket costs. Twenty-nine percent of this group had out-of-pocket costs in excess of 10 percent of their income in 1987 (Taylor and Banthin 1994).

In 1988 Congress tried to remedy the situation of lower-income elderly people by passing the Medicare Catastrophic Coverage Act, which altered the Medicare benefit package and raised premiums for higher-income beneficiaries. Higher-income beneficiaries, who already owned supplemental policies that provided many of the benefits offered by the Act, revolted. In 1989 Congress repealed the law, leaving lower-income beneficiaries to pay their own bills. The one-size-fits-all nature of the program, and the diversity of its beneficiaries, has made it difficult for Medicare to address the specific needs of lower-income elderly people.

While attempts to slash spending in Medicaid may hurt program beneficiaries, the design of the program more directly addresses the circumstances of poor people. Some state Medicaid programs cover the costs of transportation to the doctor or hospital, home care, housekeeping care for the homebound ill, hospice care, and vision care. Medicare does not provide any of these benefits; neither do most private programs (OTA 1992). Yet for a poor person, a program that pays for the costs of transportation to medical services may be more valuable—and more health improving—than one that attracts the highest-priced physicians.

Would Egalitarian Health Delivery Be Sustainable in the United States?

In most European countries, health care is explicitly "two-tiered." High-income Britons, Germans, Frenchmen, and Italians buy private insurance and use private doctors. Private insurance provides improved access to new health technology, shorter waiting lines, or more choice. In countries with an option for private insurance in the health care system, the highest-income 10 or 15 percent of the population opts for that choice (Graig 1993).

The United States is more populous and richer than these other countries, and its distribution of income is relatively more unequal (World Bank 1993). In particular, the population of high-income people in the United States is much larger than in countries with national health systems. In 1992, the income of the richest 5 percent of American households exceeded the GDP of Canada.[23] Furthermore, wealthy Americans are concentrated in a few regions of the country.

The large number and high density of wealthy Americans bodes ill for plans to generate equality by requiring everyone to participate in a centrally rationed health care system. In the New York metropolitan area in 1990, there were 667,000 households with incomes of over $100,000 U.S. (Bureau of the Census 1993a). In *all* of Canada,

530,000 families in 1990 had incomes of over $100,000 Canadian (about $85,000 U.S.; Statistics Canada 1993). Indeed, six of the ten Canadian provinces have *total* populations of fewer than 667,000 households. Wealthy U.S. communities are big enough and rich enough to support their own high-end medical technology, just as they supplement other public services available to them. Wealthy Americans send their mail by private courier, hire others to stand in line at the passport and driver's license offices, and protect their property with private security systems and private security guards.

Wealthy Americans avoid their local public school systems and in large numbers send their children to private schools. Among the highest-family-income one-third of elementary-school-aged children in the United States, fully 17 percent attend private school (Bureau of the Census 1993b).[24] This figure is all the more astonishing given the local character of public school financing in the United States.[25] Wealthy districts fund their schools much more generously than poorer ones do. The existence of a substantial population ready, willing, and quite able to buy its way around the limits of a cost-constrained public system suggests that using quantity controls in the public system as a way of limiting services and generating equality is simply unrealistic in the United States.

In the context of preexisting inequalities in American society, the complex relationship between medical care, other goods, and well-being weakens the principled arguments for strict equality in the allocation of health services. The pragmatic position that egalitarianism in health care delivery preserves the quality of care for the poor is inconsistent with the Medicaid and Medicare experience. Finally, there are just too many Americans who can afford to buy their way out of the system to imagine that a single-tier system will work. The medicalist position on health care redistribution cannot provide the basis for a successful reform.

Marketists and Redistribution

The arguments against the principle of redistributing one particular good in an egalitarian way described above apply standard neoclassical economic theory. Economists frown on programs that redistribute in-kind resources, such as health care. They argue that the goal of improving the lot of the poor could be accomplished at lower cost by simply giving the poor money. The recipients could then use the money in the way that best meets their needs. For example, today, the U.S. health care system provides very costly hospital care to homeless people and then discharges them back to the streets. The homeless would probably prefer to receive less medical care and have society spend half the savings on better housing facilities, with the rest returned to people in the form of lower taxes. Such a policy would make the homeless happier and save taxpayers money.

In the marketists' model, building on this theory, the issue of health policy can be divorced from the question of redistributing care. Society needs to decide how much money to spend on the poor. At that point the distributional question with respect to health care is best addressed the way all distributional questions ought to be addressed: by redistributing income. Once the poor have income, they can choose health care or other goods and services according to their own preferences.

The general public, however, despite years of admonitions by economists, frowns on programs that redistribute income while it (more or less) supports in-kind transfer programs. In part, this may reflect taxpayers' social concerns: if the poor get money, they may spend it on socially inappropriate goods (alcohol, drugs, movies). Given this political constraint, the next-best alternative in the marketist conception is the provision of nontransferable vouchers to the poor that they can use to buy coverage in the private health insurance market (Tobin 1970).

For marketists, the redistribution of health care is a means of redistributing income: the total amount to be redistributed is defined in dollars. Health care is the method of redistribution, not the goal, so the total amount to be redistributed depends on society's interest in income equity, not on changes in the cost or quality of health care. In a model based on income redistribution, changes in the cost of health care should lead to very little substitution of health spending for other elements of spending.

The pure marketist model calls for providing the poor with a constant dollar level of health care and other resources, a package whose size and composition varies little with changes in the quality or cost of health care. Most writers on health care policy who adhere to the marketist model, however, recognize that this pure model corresponds only weakly to the way ordinary people view health care distribution. These authors posit, instead, that the nonpoor derive benefits from knowing that poor people obtain an adequate amount of health care (Pauly 1971; Lindsay 1969). The definition of adequacy, in turn, depends on the benefits the nonpoor derive (which depend on their tastes and incomes; Pauly 1992).

In effect, this modified model, which is advocated by many, although by no means all, marketists, calls for the poor to be guaranteed a minimum bundle of health goods and services. A model of this type is the basis of the federal government's food stamp program. If the cost of purchasing the nutritionally adequate food bundle rises, food stamp allocations rise too (CBO 1977). Changes in the quality of food, or changes in middle-class preferences about food, have no effect on food stamp allocations. Only increases in the price of individual food items themselves lead to increases in the extent of redistribution.[26] In health care, a minimum-bundle model would increase payments to the poor if the price of penicillin rose, but not if a more effective but somewhat more costly treatment for infections was developed. If the minimum bundle had been specified in 1965, along with the nutritionally adequate food bundle, spending would not have risen to accommodate the cost of kidney dialysis, hip transplants, bypass surgery for heart disease, or recent innovations in chemotherapy—all lifesaving, but cost-increasing innovations that were developed since the mid-1960s (Duffy 1993).

The Effect of Changing Health Care Technology on Redistribution

As everyone knows, the United States does not have a system of universal health insurance. People without insurance coverage are guaranteed absolutely nothing by the system. Those who qualify for Medicaid may have only limited access to care. Given these miserly legal entitlements, it is remarkable how much care the poor and uninsured do receive.

The spending patterns of middle- and higher-income Americans have left the United States with a network of abundant technology, highly trained and interventionist physicians, and widespread fear of malpractice suits. Consequently, average spending among uninsured Americans, although it amounts to only 60 percent of average spending among insured Americans, is actually higher than average per capita spending in Canada, Germany, or Britain. Uninsured Americans have higher rates of use of many high-tech medical procedures than do residents of Canada, and even have higher rates of use of some low-tech preventive procedures.[27]

One recent study compared the use of heart bypass surgery for people under age sixty-five in Canada and in California as a function of income (Anderson et al. 1993). It found that low-income Canadians were as likely as or more likely than high-income Canadians to receive bypass treatment. By contrast, low-income Californians were significantly less likely to receive bypass treatment than high-income Californians. Bypass surgery is so much more frequent in California than in Canada, though, that low-income Californians were actually more likely to have bypass surgery than were Canadians of any income group.

The willingness to extend new, lifesaving procedures to the poor predates the introduction of public programs. Between 1929 and 1947, for example, philanthropic contributions to hospitals actually outpaced national health spending.[28] During the polio epidemic of the 1950s, philanthropies ensured that no one would be denied access to potentially lifesaving treatment because of a lack of money (Rothman 1993).

Poor residents of countries with more egalitarian health systems have easier access to ordinary medical care than Americans do. But in some respects, the U.S. system provides more care for its poor and uninsured members than do cost-constrained yet egalitarian systems. High-cost, high-tech procedures, used with very great frequency by privately insured Americans, do trickle down to the poor and uninsured.

The amount of care provided to poor people, whether through the Medicaid program or through uncompensated care in hospitals, is not fixed at a minimum standard, but it has risen almost as quickly as care for the nonpoor. In 1977 the average uninsured person spent half as much as the average insured person under sixty-five on health care, with just under two-thirds of these costs paid out-of-pocket.[29] In 1987, with average health care costs as a share of national income 25 percent higher, the average uninsured person again spent about half as much on health care as the average insured person. In 1987, though, only about one-third of this cost was paid out-of-pocket (Taylor and Banthin

1993). The rise in health care costs did not reduce the relative amount of care received by people without insurance. Instead, more of the cost of this care was shifted onto other payers.

Similarly, the rate of increase in Medicaid payments per beneficiary since the inception of the program has tracked, and often exceeded, the rate of increase in per capita health payments for all Americans (Reilly, Clauser, and Baugh 1990; CBO 1993c). Per capita payments for hospital services, the locus of most high-technology care, have most closely corresponded with payments for the non-Medicaid population. Attempts to reduce Medicaid costs have focused on cutting payments to providers of routine care and reducing eligibility for the program, not on limiting costly lifesaving procedures (Reilly, Clauser, and Baugh 1990).

Medicalists: Egalitarianism Matters More than High-Tech

The medicalist model demands that everyone be given an equal entitlement to health care. When rich people can get a valuable medical service, then poor people who need it must get it too. But medicalists do not demand that policymakers accommodate every improvement in health technology. If budgets are tight, medicalists prefer that the government centrally ration all health resources. Health professionals can then make allocation decisions within these constraints.

Medicalists argue for the preeminence of egalitarianism over other values in the health care system. In particular, medicalists prefer a distribution that provides equal but limited health care for all to one that provides more costly health care on average—even to the poor—but distributes that care inequitably. This position is consistent with the medicalist emphasis on professionally defined "need." An equitable distribution of basic health services will typically respond to more medically defined "needs" than an inequitable distribution of high-tech services. People may have to wait longer for new knees and hips, but they will encounter fewer obstacles in seeing a doctor when they do not feel well and in obtaining routine care.

Medicalists are willing to place severe limits on increases in costly technologies in favor of a more equitable distribution of today's health services. In this sense, medicalists need not confront the problem of adjusting health care redistribution to conform to rising health care spending. In the medicalist model, higher health spending can simply be proscribed.

Marketists: The Adequate Standard of Care

The marketist model implicitly assumes that the problem of redistribution can be solved once and for all: the amount of health care redistributed to the poor should be fixed at an adequate level and should change little over time, even as the quality of health care improves. But this model conforms weakly to American reality. Instead, health care spending for the poor has increased at about the same rate as that for higher-income Americans. As lifesaving and life-enhancing innovations are developed, they spread among the insured, the Medicaid population, and the uninsured.[30]

Marketists assert the sovereignty of individual consumption choices. Thus, the most orthodox argue against treating health care as special in any way and advocate simply redistributing income. Even those who accept the idea of redistributing health care, per se, assert that the poor should receive "adequate" care—but that the rich should be allowed to buy what they like. This model works well (given its assumptions) in many areas of policy. Americans promise poor people adequate food through the food stamp program; adequate schooling through the public education system; adequate police protection through the public law enforcement system; and, to a more limited extent, adequate shelter through housing programs. In each case, poor people receive some politically defined minimum standard of these goods and higher-income people buy what they want.

Improvements in the quality of food eaten by middle-class people, in the schools they attend, in the security of their homes, or in the housing they live in have had limited effects on the extent of redistribution of these goods and services to the poor. Quality changes in these other entitlements have been quite slow. Health care is different. The frequent changes in health services use among the well-to-do translate directly into changes in the health services provided to the poor. When no one received heart transplants, poor people did not receive them. Once the technology became available to the well-to-do, it was almost immediately diffused to the poor, albeit at lower usage rates (Thurow 1984).

The pattern of redistribution in health care reflects the peculiar nature of American attitudes toward medicine. Although marketists and medicalists alike decry such attitudes, Americans seem much more willing to pay to rescue a child from a well, or to pay for high-technology care for a dying patient, than they are to pay for preventive care, auto safety, or income redistribution. Faced with the stark possibility that someone will die for lack of medical care, society provides that care. Even if the minimum standard defined in a benefit package included only care that would appreciably and immediately reduce that person's risk of dying, the constantly improving health technologies, which are freely selected by higher-income Americans, would translate into more costly care for the poor. A hospital that does not stock costly treatment for patients with myocardial infarction cannot provide them to a poor person. Once the hospital stocks the treatment for higher-income people, it is unlikely to deny it to the poor.[31]

Redistribution, whether of health care or of income, does have efficiency implications. After all, if people do not have to pay for their own medical care, they have less incentive to work. At the moment of a life-or-death decision (although not before), Americans seem willing to put aside these efficiency implications. Even the most hardheaded marketist would open the hospital doors for a patient who could be immediately saved from death using a technology inside that hospital. This minimal level of egalitarianism, though, is enough to ruin the marketist conception of redistribution. As health technologies improve, more and more people on the steps of the hospital can be saved using the technologies inside.

The marketist model of redistribution fails to address the interrelatedness of health care decisions. When private-pay patients choose to use more resources, the call on government and philanthropists to fund care also increases. The experience of the uninsured suggests that the effects of private health spending are not translated exclusively through government programs. Those without any insurance coverage receive much less treatment than do those with coverage; but they receive substantial amounts of care. The uninsured are 50 to 70 percent less likely than similarly situated insured people to receive most non-lifesaving high-tech services. The uninsured are just as likely as the insured to receive low-discretion, lifesaving treatment (OTA 1992).

A pattern in which increasing health costs among higher-income

Americans lead to a rising call on public coffers poses problems in the marketist model. The medicalist model avoids the potential effects of improved technology on the cost of redistribution by arbitrarily capping spending for everyone. The marketist model rejects this approach, arguing that consumers alone should decide what health care they want to buy. This rejection, though, leaves marketists with two alternatives. The increasing call on public spending may mean ever rising taxes and ever rising distortionary effects on the economy: the experience of the Medicare hospital insurance program. Alternatively, the increased need to buy health for the poor may mean cuts in other, more beneficial programs.[32] Marketists dislike both outcomes.

Policies governing the distribution of health resources to the poor differ from other redistributive policies. Polling results suggest that most Americans believe, in principle, that health care should be distributed equitably (although they are reluctant to pay the price). Health care in the United States is certainly not distributed equally today, but the poor receive more equitable treatment with respect to health care than with respect to most other goods. Yet treating all health care as special, as medicalists suggest, means subsidizing people who seek medical interventions for their problems, without providing comparable assistance to people with similar conditions who prefer nonmedical treatment.

The superior ability of the medical model to describe public attitudes points to a principal flaw in the market model of health care as it confronts ever improving health technologies. Although the market model argues that individual spending decisions should be respected, the empirical evidence indicates that decisions to increase spending among the insured also affect the care of the uninsured. The market model fails to account for this reality.

Neither the medicalist nor the marketist model passes the reality test with respect to redistribution. The medicalist model captures Americans' idealistic attitudes about redistribution, but its prescription of constrained overall spending and limits on what the wealthy can buy for themselves are both undesirable in theory and unsustainable in practice. Americans want more health care, not less, and the sheer numbers and wealth of higher-income Americans would make it almost impossible to keep them within a tightly constrained system. Marketists would permit health care technology to grow unbridled, but at the same time would require that new and effective technology be denied to those who cannot readily afford it. That disheartening prescription violates Americans stated preferences and conforms poorly to their observed behavior. American health care financing has not explicitly accommodated the costs of improved health care technology, but in actual practice that technology has been disseminated nonetheless.

6 ///

The Institutional Structure of Reform

Health care reform proposals should be judged by how well the institutional structures they establish cope with the dynamic nature of health care—the constancy of change. A successful health reform will provide a framework that accommodates and encourages efficiency-enhancing reforms, conserves government funds, and guarantees that the fruits of change are spread among all Americans. Unfortunately, most health reform plans focus on the here and now, proposing solutions that provide immediate relief but do not stem long-term deterioration.[1]

The Structure of Medicalist Reform

Canada

Among medicalists, the conventional wisdom is that the optimal design for national health coverage is a single-payer plan modeled on Canada's health care system. More than any other plan, a single-payer model would assure universal coverage and equity in health delivery and would eliminate concerns over health security. Technically, a single-payer plan, in which all money comes from one spigot, could be designed to save any amount of money. Spending could be reduced to the desired level by simply turning off the tap.

In a Canadian-style single-payer system, the government (in Canada, the ten provincial governments) pays all medical bills.[2] Physicians are paid on a fee-for-service basis with fees set by the payer. Hospitals are paid using global budgets—that is, annual funding streams negotiated each year with the payer. Private citizens cannot purchase alternative health insurance and providers cannot charge patients any out-of-pocket cost (balance billing). Patients pay little or nothing as coinsurance or deductibles. As the sole purchaser, the government can exercise its market power to keep prices low.

Medicalists argue that the Clinton administration's failure to put forward a single-payer plan reflected a bow to political realities rather than policy rationales (Marmor 1994). Many members of the Clinton administration did favor a single-payer plan, but many others had principled reasons for preferring alternatives.

The 1980s were the heyday of policy interest in the Canadian model. Earlier reformers had lauded the merits of the British health care system, a more restrictive model in which all health care providers are employed directly by the government (Stevens and Stevens 1974). The Canadian health care system loosened some of the constraints of the British model. Rather than nationalizing the provision of care by hiring doctors and taking over hospitals, Canada retained private provision of care. Pollsters find that Canadians like their health system much more than Americans like their own system (Graig 1993).

The Canadian single-payer model, with its single tier of health provision and prohibition of balance billing is very egalitarian. Furthermore, the quality of medical care is very high. Despite allegations of rationing, Canada is second only to the United States in its per capita endowment of costly technology. As advocates of the system point out, administrative costs are very low (OECD 1993a). Doctors and hospitals employ many fewer administrative staff than do their U.S. counterparts and the government processes claims at low cost (GAO 1992b). During the 1970s, Canadian health care spending as a share of GDP hardly budged (Glied 1993).

In the late 1980s, though, analysts began to question the strengths of the Canadian system. By 1990 the three wealthiest English-speaking provinces, Ontario, Alberta, and British Columbia, began sending patients to the United States to alleviate waiting lists for heart bypass surgery (President 1992; Graig 1993). A 1991 report identified queues for 47 out of the 48 elective surgical procedures considered; some queues were as long as a year (GAO 1992b). Many of the queues were short lived, but they lasted long enough—and received enough publicity—to be politically salient (Marmor 1994). More important to many cost cutters, real per capita health care costs were growing almost as quickly in Canada as in the United States.[3] Despite low administrative costs and virtually complete control over doctors' fees, hospital expenditures, health capital, and pharmaceutical prices, Canada has the second-most-expensive health system in the world after the United States and, especially prior to recent severe budget cuts, has experienced growth rates in cost that are quite close to U.S. per capita growth rates.

Canadian health care costs are substantially lower than U.S. costs, so that the absolute size of the gap between U.S. and Canadian costs has been widening. But governments bear a much larger share of those costs in Canada than in the United States, and federal and provincial revenues have not kept pace with escalating health care costs. The budgetary consequences of the Canadian health system have been nothing short of disastrous. Indeed, more than anything else, the impact of Canada's health insurance system on its budget tempered the enthusiasm of cost-conscious reformers. In recent polls Canadians, too, have begun to question the strength of their health care system (Blendon et al. 1995).

In 1992 the portion of Canadian provincial government deficits attributable primarily to the costs of the health care system amounted to $19.4 billion Canadian, or 2.8 percent of Canadian GDP (OECD 1993a).[4] Canada's combined budget deficit (federal, provincial, and local) in fiscal year 1992–93 exceeded 5 percent of national GDP (Canada Health 1993). By contrast, the combined U.S. deficit (including all levels of government) for 1993 amounted to 2.5 percent of U.S. GDP (CEA 1995). In 1993 Ontario, Canada's wealthiest province, ran a budget deficit of $17 billion Canadian ($13 billion U.S.; Ontario 1993). On a per capita basis this provincial deficit was 35 percent higher than the U.S. federal deficit.[5]

In response to these deficits, provincial governments have taken ever more restrictive steps to constrain spending. In 1993 Ontario proposed real fee cuts, closure of more hospital beds (16 percent of beds were closed between 1990 and 1993), limits on the number of new doctors who could practice in the province, experiments in moving away from fee-for-service billing, closer monitoring of fraud, and efforts to encourage older doctors to retire (Ontario 1993). For 1995 the government went even further, proposing to monitor the services physicians provide and reserving the right to withhold payment for unnecessary services (Ontario Ministry 1994).

These changes are likely to cool provider support for single-payer reform in the United States. While most physicians have always opposed such a reform, a surprising number of the key supporters of a single-payer plan in the most recent reform debates have been physicians (Berenson 1994). The growing role of insurance contracts with managed-care features has generated a backlash among physicians, who complain that insurers today are eroding traditional physician autonomy. Under a single-payer system, they argue, doctors practice medicine as they wish and someone else worries about its cost.

This faith in physician autonomy under national health insurance is misplaced. As Canadian physicians are discovering, national health insurance systems, like private insurers, must somehow control the volume of services provided. Despite the hubbub over physician oversight by insurers in the United States, physicians in other countries also lament their loss of professional autonomy. A recent survey of physicians in Canada, Germany, and the United States found that all physicians have reasons to complain—the reasons just differ. Canadian physicians griped loudest about limitations on the availability of services. Germans complained the most about administrative burdens and bureaucracy and about not having enough time to spend with each patient. American physicians protested that their patients could not afford treatment and that they had trouble receiving payment because of disputes in processing insurance forms (Blendon et al. 1993). Complete physician autonomy in medical-practice decisions is simply incompatible with third-party payment mechanisms, whether the third-party is a private insurance company or the state.

Germany

In the late 1980s, analysts concerned with the fiscal implications of health policy turned their attention from Canada toward Germany. Between 1984 and 1990, Germany had achieved the almost impossible: it held real per capita health care costs almost steady.[6] Germany's system is so complex that it makes the final Clinton plan look (almost) simple.

More than 1,200 private insurers, called sickness funds, cover most Germans. A small minority, about 10 percent, are covered by private insurance that is not regulated by sickness fund rules and that provides somewhat enhanced access to specialists and hospital services (GAO 1993b). Sickness funds negotiate fees with local physicians' unions, which oversee the volume of care provided by individual doctors. The success of the German system, with its amalgam of private insurance, strict regulation, and cooperative behavior encouraged renewed interest in health reform models with multiple payers. Even Germany, though, has had problems controlling spending. Despite continuing restrictions on fees and utilization, the payroll tax rates needed to fund the sickness funds increased by 1 percentage point between 1991 and 1992—prompting still another round of "emergency" belt-tightening reforms (GAO 1993b).

Despite its fiscal savings, the German model, with its disparities of insurance coverage between rich and poor, did not appeal to strict egalitarians. The highly interventionist local physicians' unions, which ensure that utilization does not exceed sickness fund targets, annoyed physicians. In addition, the high administrative costs and complexity of the German system appalled those who argued that administrative costs were the scourge of the U.S. system. As a result, Canada has remained the model for most medicalists.

Problems in the Medicalist Institutional Structure: Responses to Regulation

The rapid increase in Canadian health care costs seems inconsistent with the highly centralized and regulated nature of the system. The discrepancy between apparently stringent controls on spending and concrete increases in costs occurs because of the ways that actors within the systems have responded to its constraints. Such responses are endemic to regulatory institutional structures.

The case of Canadian doctors, who have managed to maintain relatively high income levels despite 20 years of fee controls, illustrates the nature of regulatory response. As in the U.S. Medicare system, Canadian provincial payers control physician costs almost entirely through limits on fees. Between 1971 and 1981, real fee schedules for Canadian physicians fell 22 percent (Barer, Evans, and Labelle 1985). Physician incomes, however, hardly declined. Consistent with the Medicare experience, physicians offset the dip in fees by increasing the volume of patient visits.[7] The average number of visits per patient increased 50 percent and the average number of visits per physician increased 13 percent (Glied 1993). The huge increase in volume compensated for the loss in fees, and between 1971 and 1980, real physician billings per capita rose almost 2 percent per year.

This explosion in volume mainly represented physician response to the declining fee schedule. Prior to reforms in the system in 1984, Canadian physicians could charge patients amounts above those mandated by the fee schedule, a practice called opting out. A study of opting-out physicians in Ontario described practice patterns that more closely resemble those of pre-reform (or U.S.) physicians. Opting-out physicians had fewer visits each day and provided more services at each visit (Wolfson and Tuohy 1980).

Just as physicians adjusted the volume of services they rendered to compensate for cuts in fees, Canadian hospitals have responded to the incentives they face. Under global hospital budgets, Canadian hospitals have no incentive to shorten length of stay. By keeping beds full of low-cost recovering patients, they can retain their budgets for future years while keeping costs down (Evans et al. 1989).

These responses to regulation make the work of regulators more difficult and the potential savings from regulation harder to achieve. They also increase unmeasured patient costs: patients make more unnecessary physician visits and also spend unnecessary time in the hospital. Better estimates of the scope and magnitude of such regulatory responses have strengthened the case against regulation as a means of cost control. Still, by constantly adjusting the rules governing payment, regulators can compensate for these behaviors. For example, the failure to control physician spending has spurred more and more control on the volume of physician services in Canada. Rather than controlling services directly, provinces have limited physicians' earnings, restricted practice opportunities in big cities, and encouraged retirement of physicians over sixty-five (Lomas et al. 1989). Of course, these efforts also lead to provider responses. Reports from Quebec suggest that some physicians just shut their offices and go on vacation when they reach the cap level (Graig 1993).

Regulators find it especially difficult to adjust to changes in the underlying technology of health care delivery and to alter the structure of delivery. In many respects, the structure of health care delivery in Canada is petrified in the form it had in the late 1960s, before comprehensive insurance was introduced. Physicians' associations and existing hospitals, which bargain with provincial payers to set fee schedules, have proved resistant to changes that would diminish their effectiveness.

The most obvious difference between the institutions of medical practice in the United States and Canada is the relative absence of integrated delivery and group practice in Canada (Kissick 1994). By 1990, 33 million Americans (more than the population of Canada) were receiving care through HMOs (CEA 1993). In the United States, group practices have flourished, providing a way for doctors to share capital, support staff, and expertise; to build a patient base through the reputation of the group; and to negotiate with third parties. A recent study finds that doctors in group practices have lower expenses of practice than do solo practitioners (Dynan 1994).

While HMOs and group practices have prospered in the United States, almost all Canadian doctors continue to work in small fee-for-service practices. The few community-based practices that had existed before the coming of provincial health insurance have had trouble surviving (Roemer and Roemer 1977).

There are no incentives to form or join HMOs in Canada. The cost savings of HMOs yield no benefits to either doctors or patients. Physicians have limited support staff and little incentive to invest in capital. Without third-party payers, the negotiating function of group practices is reduced. Restrictions on generating profit from medical practice limit the ability of groups to develop efficient fee-sharing schemes.

Patients pay no copayments or deductibles even under fee-for-service practice in Canada. There are no premiums, so they receive no premium savings by choosing a lower-cost plan. Medical associations strongly resist efforts to encourage the formation of clinic-style practices (as they did in the United States), but since consumers cannot gain financially by choosing these clinics, they have little incentive to lobby for their formation.

The provincial governments have little reason to press for the growth of capitated practices. Operating both a capitated and a fee-for-service system at once poses complex problems. As the U.S. Medicare system has found, if people who are attracted to HMOs differ from those who choose fee-for-service providers, payments may overcompensate (or undercompensate) HMOs (Brown et al. 1993). Running two distinct payment systems at once more than doubles bureaucratic headaches: not only must regulators set prices in two systems, but they must ensure that the prices correctly relate to each other.

Medicalists laud the single-payer system for eliminating cost from any provider's decision about what care to provide. But the absence of cost-consciousness has its downside. Entrepreneurial incentives to develop new ways of delivering care more efficiently have been closed off. The lack of economic incentives limits the likelihood of integrated delivery of health care. Physician payments are independent of payments to hospitals, so neither physicians nor hospitals consider the relative cost of inpatient and outpatient treatment in making allocation decisions in individual cases. The lack of integrated delivery and third-party oversight also makes diffusion of changes in medical practice more difficult. Each physician must independently monitor changes in scientific knowledge and innovations that require investment in capital must be centrally coordinated.

In the hospital sector, the influence of established providers in slowing change can be seen in the lack of decline in length of stay. In 1970 average length of stay in Canada was the same as in the United States (OECD 1993b). In 1989, though, the average length of stay in short-stay hospitals in Ontario was 8.2 days, compared with an average of 6.6 days in the United States (DHHS 1993; Ontario 1994). Since then, massive government-mandated bed cutbacks led to a substantial and very rapid decline in length of stay. By 1993 length of stay in Ontario had fallen to 6.5 days, marginally above the U.S. level in 1992.

The slower change in Canada can be attributed, in part, to a failure to establish freestanding diagnostic and surgical facilities. In the United States, most of these facilities were started by profit-hungry entrepreneurs. Canadian entrepreneurs could not expect comparable opportunities for profit within the health care system. Instead, a small number of private, for-profit freestanding clinics in Canada opened outside the national health care system. They accept only cash payments and receive no funding from the government. One private freestanding facility in Alberta, the Gimbel Clinic, does 5 percent of all the cataract surgery in Canada (Graig 1993). Another, the Shouldice Clinic in Ontario, pioneered the development of outpatient treatment for hernias. Operating outside the bounds of the health care system, these private providers responded to the development of new surgical techniques much more quickly than did the national system.

Political Impediments to Change

Single-payer systems provide no incentives, in money or extra services, for either physicians or patients to choose less costly alternatives. Without these incentives, all adjustments aimed at reducing cost must come through regulatory decisions. Regulatory control, however, is not only technically difficult but also politically difficult because consumers and providers are allied in their determination to retain existing services and facilities.

As in the U.S. Medicare program (which is also a single-payer plan), cutbacks in Canadian health care have, until quite recently, focused entirely on reductions in the pay of doctors and hospitals. Regulators hoped that stringent price controls alone would eliminate the need for explicit supply-control policies. Canadian provincial governments had always required that health facilities obtain approval for new investments in technological equipment. Now, under continuing fiscal pressure, provincial governments have begun to close and consolidate existing facilities.

Centralized control over resources raises two politically unpleasant specters. From a public relations perspective, having the government restrict access to existing technology smacks of rationing, and such methods are rarely invoked. Within legislatures, health planning threatens to pit communities against one another, generating the same sort of political heat that military-base closings do. Health planning is much more popular among politicians when it involves building capacity than when it involves reducing it.

At the same time, if regulators set prices, they must decide what to do when the prices do not suffice to support an existing facility. Planning the number of health care facilities requires a continual balancing of conflicting political and policy factors. This balancing act favors existing facilities, with established constituencies, over new, unknown entrants. A vocal and politically intimidating constituency of local consumers, politicians, and providers is likely to oppose closings, while no general constituency will arise to support cutbacks or transfers of funds to new facilities. Health facility planning may be moderately successful in creating completely new resources; it is almost certain to disappoint in attempts to rationalize the existing stock.

If anything, the political difficulties of sustaining fiscal stability under a single-payer program would be more difficult in the United States than in Canada. Canada's highly centralized parliamentary system makes it easier for the government to take actions that hurt powerful lobby groups. In the United States, stringent reductions in pay to doctors and hospitals and direct controls on technology would encounter even stiffer opposition, as well as a complex process of regulatory oversight (Fossett 1994).[8] Canadians are well aware of their advantage. The deputy minister of health in Ontario, Martin Barkin, complained in 1992 of "the 'Americanization of Canadian parliamentary democracy,' " and "the increasing role of the Charter of Rights [Canada's version of the Bill of Rights], the courts and lobby groups"—forces that increasingly require the government to build consensus using advisory structures and other more open mechanisms (Barkin 1992, p. 5). Barkin noted that "by their very nature these mechanisms are slow, whereas the pace of change [in health care] . . . is fast" (ibid., p. 6).

Previous attempts to limit reimbursement for specific services within the U.S. Medicare program illustrate the effects of this problem. In one case, it took seven years to withdraw coverage for a treatment, thermography, although two separate studies had recommended this action (Buto 1994). Use of another discredited technology, intermittent positive pressure breathing, declined much more rapidly among patients of private payers than among those of public payers.[9]

The development and strengthening of consumer-side lobby groups in the United States during the 1980s further undermines the ability of a government-run system to make rational health planning decisions. Prior to the 1980s, providers had been the most powerful health lobbyists. During the eighties, the lobbying balance changed. The American Medical Association, the principal physicians' association, grew weaker, in part because competition for the business of managed-care plans pitted physicians against one another. Hospitals, too, began to negotiate directly with insurers, leading to conflicts between hospitals about price.

Meanwhile, health care consumer lobbies gained strength. Consumer lobbies, including the American Red Cross and the American Cancer Society, had always been powerful. Before the 1980s, though, consumer groups of this type had focused on increasing appropriations for research (Rettig 1994). In the 1980s, these consumer lobbies began to challenge reimbursement policies. Two lobby groups, the AARP and ACT UP, transformed the role of lobbies in health care policy making.

The AARP rose to prominence in health policy during the catastrophic-coverage debate. The original Medicare program left beneficiaries uninsured for catastrophic illnesses and pharmaceuticals. In 1988 Congress passed a bill designed to protect Medicare beneficiaries from the risk of catastrophic illness and give them coverage for prescription drugs. The bill would have required Medicare beneficiaries to pay a higher premium to receive these benefits. It would also have imposed a tax on the Medicare benefits of higher-income Medicare beneficiaries. The bill, viewed as good policy by a majority of Democrats and Republicans, and supported by almost all health care policy wonks and by the AARP, passed resoundingly.

A number of higher-income older people, however, objected to the Catastrophic Act and marshaled substantial grass-roots opposition. Medicare beneficiaries felt that it was unfair for them to bear the entire cost of enhanced Medicare coverage. Higher-income beneficiaries, who already had catastrophic-type coverage and prescription coverage through supplemental policies, gained nothing from passage of the Catastrophic Act, but were required to pay higher premiums and taxes to pay for it.

Opposition to the act grew. The elderly marched on Washington and threw eggs at House Ways and Means Committee chairman Dan Rostenkowski's car. In 1989 Congress repealed the Catastrophic Act, again by an overwhelming margin. All but one senator who had supported the original bill backed its repeal.

The Catastrophic catastrophe shook Congress. Any prospects for revising Medicare that cut benefits or increased costs for existing beneficiaries would be viewed with enormous skepticism. If the cost of Medicare was to be pared, cuts would have to come from providers. The cost of estranging the provider lobby did not even remotely approach the cost of enraging the elderly.

Congress's fear of the elderly lobby survived the 1994 congressional elections. Of the $270 billion in Medicare savings proposed by the

House the following year, only 20 percent came from increases in premiums paid by elderly beneficiaries (CBO 1995).[10]

The AIDS lobby resembles more traditional health care lobbying groups in that its interest in the health system is disease-specific. The lobby's primary goal is to increase government spending on AIDS research. It has also, though, focused on changing the Food and Drug Administration's policies for testing new drugs and has lobbied successfully to have AIDS classified as a disabling condition under the Social Security Act, thereby making people with AIDS eligible for Medicare (Rettig 1994). Later, the lobby pressed to broaden the definition of AIDS and, thus, the number of people who would qualify for Medicare (House Committee 1992).

AIDS activists operated through a broad public campaign rather than relying on a few well-placed congressional insiders to advance their cause. Their success has led other groups to use similar strategies. A new lobbying paradigm has been established. For example, breast cancer activists have successfully lobbied to require the federal employees' health program to cover experimental autologous bone marrow transplant treatment (Rettig 1994). People who require treatment for an illness, especially costly treatment for a very serious illness, now demand a response from Congress. Faced with a small but vocal single-issue constituency made up of people willing to chain themselves to buildings to get their point across, politicians are likely to expand coverage for that narrow group. Larger, less well-organized groups are likely to be ignored.

The U.S. political system may impede attempts at private-sector cost containment too. Patient advocates have also succeeded in expanding the generosity of health spending outside Congress. Those with private insurance coverage increasingly use the legal system to expand the range of treatments made available to them. Most insurance contracts specifically disallow coverage for experimental treatments. Juries, though, have proved resistant to contract provisions that limit care to patients whose life is on the line (Aaron 1993). "Any willing provider" laws and patient protection acts limit managed-care firms' ability to control costs by selecting low-cost providers.[11] The federal government, following the lead of many states, has adopted legislation mandating that all health plans provide coverage for 48-hour hospital stays after childbirth (the Newborns' and Mothers' Health Protection Act of 1996). All of these developments restrict the ability of private-sector health providers to reduce the cost of care.

The Structure of Marketist Reform

Medicalists place enormous faith in the ability of health regulators to make sensible allocation decisions. They argue that markets have failed in health care and that a government-run program is the only reasonable alternative. Marketists, although divided among themselves about the direction for further reform, argue that the market has not really been tried yet. They propose a range of reforms centered around eliminating inefficiencies in the market that lead consumers to make health care choices without concern for their costs.

Marketists agree that the effects of moral hazard are the most important source of efficiency problems in the health sector. This emphasis presupposes a very different vision of efficiency than that implicit in medicalist designs. Efficiency, in the marketist model, does not necessarily mean that all resources are used to full capacity at every point in time, nor that the earnings of heart surgeons do not zoom up 30 percent in a decade, nor that insurers never fail. Many of the marks of inefficiency in the medicalist model are simply beside the point in the marketist model.

Where medicalists emphasize the comparison of static costs and benefits, examining the cost-effectiveness of particular technologies or the payments associated with some particular set of physician skills, marketists focus on the underlying structure of incentives within the system. In an unfettered market, one with minimal government intervention, incentives will be appropriately aligned. Short-run departures from efficiency in such a market are just steps on the road toward an eventual equilibrium.

The most straightforward marketist approach is reform of the tax subsidy for health insurance combined with insurance vouchers (such as refundable tax credits; Pauly et al. 1992). Under this plan, the existing open-ended tax subsidy for health insurance purchase would be replaced by a flat credit or voucher that would have to be used toward the purchase of a health plan. All health plans sold would have to include a basic level of benefits, but insurers could offer additional features. Plan prices would not be regulated (and most would, presumably, exceed the voucher level).

The voucher plan's centerpiece—replacement of the tax subsidy with a better-designed incentive for health insurance purchase—is also central to the design of the best-known marketist approach, managed competition. Developed in the 1970s, managed competition is a formulation that responds logically to each of the economic problems of the health care market in turn, with elements intended to minimize the effects of moral hazard, adverse selection, asymmetric information, and provider market power (Enthoven 1993).

The voucher plan builds on economists' long-standing complaint that the tax subsidy aggravates the effects of moral hazard in the market by leading people to buy coverage with low deductibles and limited coinsurance. The designers of managed competition focused particularly on the role of the tax subsidy in slowing the growth of HMOs. HMO supporters traced consumer reluctance to join these plans to a lack of cost-consciousness. Consumers choosing plans placed little value on low cost, they argued, so HMOs found it most profitable to offer very generous benefits and keep their prices only slightly lower than the prices of fee-for-service plans.

Empirical evidence suggests that traditional HMOs, which limit patients to a fixed panel of capitated providers, have the capacity to reduce costs by as much as 25 percent relative to fee-for-service plans with similar copayments and deductibles (Luft 1978; Newhouse 1993a). Nonetheless, most HMO plans charged almost the same premiums as fee-for-service plans. Employers switching to HMOs typically saw their premium costs increase rather than decrease as they loaded plans with features that would please their employees.

HMO supporters, like the voucher plan group, blame this lack of cost-consciousness on inadequacies in the health market, such as the tax subsidy for employer-provided health insurance. The tax subsidy, together with the common employer practice of paying a constant proportion of health insurance premiums, they felt, insulated consumers from the costs of coverage. Like voucher proponents, they sought to make consumers bear more of the incremental costs of coverage themselves.

The managed-competition group, however, went further than

voucher plan supporters. Cost-conscious choice alone, they argued, might not make the health care market competitive. Insurers would continue to have an incentive to dilute the unobservable quality of plans to lure consumers. Adverse selection would continue as low-risk consumers chose less generous plans. Physicians would continue to retain the cartel power conferred by state licensing boards. Eliminating the tax subsidy alone could not solve all these problems.

Instead, the managed-competition group developed a model that blended competitive and regulatory elements (Enthoven 1993). The plan proposes that the health insurance tax subsidy be limited to the price of the lowest-cost health plan in a region and that employers make equal premium contributions to any plan their employees choose. It establishes a standard benefit package that each insurer must offer and stipulates that insurers must take all comers during annual open-enrollment periods and may not impose preexisting-condition clauses. Finally, it mandates that each participating insurer be certified as meeting uniform quality standards and regularly report measures of quality assurance as well as disenrollment statistics.

Standard benefits, certified insurers, and quality assurance measures are intended to provide consumers with the information they need to assess and compare plans. Consumers already face the full marginal cost of differences in health plan quality, since pain and suffering cannot be insured. Under the managed-competition plan, they could trade-off the marginal value and marginal cost of quality differences among plans.

Voucher plan supporters argue that much of the superstructure of managed competition is unnecessary (Pauly et al. 1992). Other, more conservative analysts find managed competition alarming because of the emphasis it places on managed care. Managed competition would eliminate current policies that promote the purchase of costly coverage and, therefore, would likely lead more consumers to choose managed care voluntarily.[12]

Rather than eliminating the tax subsidy, some marketists would extend it further, protecting from taxes payments made into medical savings accounts as well as purchases of health insurance. Medical savings accounts, patterned after individual retirement accounts, would permit the tax-free accumulation of savings that could be used to pay deductible and copayment amounts associated with health care use and could be rolled over from year to year. Funds in medical savings accounts could be used to pay routine expenditures. Catastrophic costs would be paid through either privately purchased or government-provided catastrophic insurance coverage.

There is no consensus among marketists about which of these paths is the right one to follow. Managed-competition and medical-savings-account proponents are at loggerheads. Voucher plan supporters do not much like medical savings accounts either. They argue that these accounts distort choice away from managed-care plans, which may be at least as good at eliminating moral hazard. By expanding the tax subsidy, medical savings accounts would also further extend the federal government's exposure to rising health care costs.

Marketists of whatever stripe contend that by relying on the market they can avoid the centralized allocation problems and special-interest lobbying that would mark a single-payer plan. To the extent possible, they eliminate government from the functioning of their plans. Marketists concede, though, that the unencumbered market will not provide much care to the poor (because they cannot afford it) or coverage at reasonable prices to people who have already become ill (because of the problems associated with adverse selection). All the marketist reform plans rely on the government to complete the work of the market.

Problems with the Marketist Model: Standardizing Benefits

All marketist plans turn to regulation to combat problems of selection in insurance markets. Marketist plans recognize that adverse selection (and risk selection) may persist, indeed may be enhanced, in a market where consumers face the full cost of their health care choices. Some marketist plans propose to use risk adjustment mechanisms to address this problem, but use of these mechanisms requires a significant amount of intervention in the health insurance market. The least regulatory way to avoid the most serious effects of adverse selection, a method adopted by most plans, is to set a minimum standard benefit package that everyone must purchase.

A minimum benefit package serves two functions. First, it provides a benchmark for vouchers. Second, by mandating coverage at a minimum level, marketist plans can avoid the complete disintegration of the market that can occur if adverse selection operates unchecked. No one, however healthy, could buy a plan less generous than the minimum.

Beyond the *minimum* benefit package, proponents of managed competition would require that all benefit packages sold include only a single, defined set of benefits. This would facilitate consumer shopping and reduce adverse selection effects further. Many marketists favor the selection of a moral-hazard-moderating minimum benefit package with relatively high deductible and coinsurance levels.

Standardizing benefits seems straightforward, but taking even this first step away from the free market creates problems within the marketist model. Simply by specifying and guaranteeing a minimum benefit package, the marketist model sacrifices some of its superior ability to respond to change. Any attempt to standardize benefits will retard innovation in the design of benefit packages. For example, had the standard benefit packages been chosen six or seven years ago, they probably would not have included point-of-service plans. Furthermore, standardizing benefits exposes the marketist model to the problems of regulatory cost containment that plague the single-payer plan.

Standardization of benefits requires the politically torturous determination of what constitutes a basic benefit package. As the range of plan types proliferates, this exercise becomes increasingly difficult. Combinations of coinsurance and deductibles with an assortment of managed care features make the problem dizzying. Reformers must also define the scope of standardization: Does a plan that offers elective surgery only after a one-year delay qualify as a minimum benefit plan?

Once standards have been set and the profusion of existing plans limited to a few generic types, reformers must address the problem of benefit supplementation, allowing consumers to buy plans that supplement the standard benefits. Prohibiting supplementation reduces consumer choice and, as the Clinton administration discovered, increases the difficulties of mandating a benefit package. But allowing supplementation generates its own problems. If the government pays for coverage at some minimum standard, the value of that coverage can be enhanced through the purchase of complementary coverage. In the Canadian single-payer system, for example, people purchase private-room insurance for their hospital stays, enhancing the value of their government-provided medical coverage.

In the United States, the effects of subsidized, high-deductible coverage combined with supplementation can be seen in the Medicare program. The basic Medicare package has relatively high deductibles and coinsurance. Although its cost-sharing levels may be too high for those with low incomes, as a middle-class package it might satisfy most marketists. In practice, though, few beneficiaries actually face these deductibles. Over two-thirds of Medicare beneficiaries have private Medigap insurance (PROPAC 1993). Since 1990 government regulations have required that all Medigap policies sold cover most coinsurance expenses.[13] Even before passage of these regulations, though, beneficiaries favored up-front coverage (especially of hospital expenses). Cost-sharing Medigap coverage enhances the value to purchasers of their existing Medicare entitlement. Beneficiaries with cost-sharing coverage use substantially more services than do those without such coverage (Christensen, Long, and Rodgers 1987). After the deductibles and co-payments have been paid, the remainder of the cost of these services is reimbursed by the Medicare program.

The cost of the Medigap policy, though, includes only the cost of deductibles and copayments that will be paid through that policy, not the additional Medicare payments that will be made because of Medigap. For example, a person might decline a $500 procedure if she has to pay $100 of the cost as a copayment. With the copayment covered by Medigap, though, she will go ahead with the procedure. Her Medigap premium only accounts for the $100 copayment expense. The full cost of the coverage includes the additional $400 in Medicare spending. Estimates of this effect of Medigap coverage suggest that it raises total Medicare spending by 24 percent over the amount that would be spent if no such coverage were available (ibid.). Thus Medigap policies provide two benefits to purchasers: they reduce up-front risk and they increase the value of Medicare. The price of the policies, though, incorporates only the first of these benefits; the second comes free of charge.[14]

In completely unregulated markets without subsidies or basic government-provided packages, people would not supplement their health plans. Those who wanted policies with more generous coinsurance and deductible provisions could purchase such policies directly.[15] When the government limits the number of available plans, though, supplementation can generate undesirable outcomes. The unregulated sale of supplemental coverage can have the perverse effect of driving out of the market the very policies with high deductibles and coinsurance most favored by marketists.[16] The price of frequently supplemented policies will increase to reflect the cost of the supplementation-induced extra utilization. This rise in costs, in turn, may lead people who would have preferred an unsupplemented plan to purchase supplementation. If the government provides vouchers or subsidies tied to the cost of the basic plan, it will find that cost rising even without changes in health services.

The trade-off between the political benefits of permitting free supplementation and the economic costs of doing so became apparent in discussions of supplementation within the Clinton task force. To keep costs down, the fee-for-service benefit package proposed by the task force would have had moderately high deductibles and coinsurance for most services. Roughly 80 percent of the fee-for-service benefit plans purchased by employees of large firms had lower coinsurance rates. In order to retain political support from unions, the administration proposed permitting employers to supplement the health plans by paying deductibles and coinsurance on behalf of their employees. Since all employees of all firms would pay the same price for each health plan, this arrangement would have increased the value of the fee-for-service plan to employees of firms that supplemented benefits. Employees of supplementing firms might pay the full cost of the deductibles and coinsurance, but they would not pay the full cost of the additional utilization. That cost would be spread among all purchasers of the fee-for-service plan.[17]

The supplementation problem can be solved by limiting or regulating the kinds of supplementation that accompany the basic benefit package. Supplemental cost-sharing coverage could be priced to include the full cost to the health system of that gap-filling coverage. Alternatively, insurers could be restricted to selling cost-sharing coverage only to those who purchase standard benefits through their plan. Such regulations reduce choice in the market and add to the political heat of designing a benefit package, but without them, cost-sharing coverage will proliferate in the standard health insurance market as it has in the Medicare market, eliminating the ability to control volume through cost sharing.

Overseeing the System

Plans that promise universal health coverage, even those that rely heavily on markets, require additional oversight authority. Someone has to ensure that insurance plans offering benefits at the voucher level are indeed available, that benefits meet the requirements of minimum standards, that supplemental coverage is sold only under appropriate conditions, and that people at high risk can obtain affordable coverage. When insurers fail, as undoubtedly some will in a well-functioning market, someone has to guarantee continuation of coverage through other plans.

In an undiluted market, these tasks could be left in private hands and consumers could be left to fend for themselves. Even in the purest marketist conception, however, the reformed health market differs from this ideal in two respects. First, the government already has a role in the market because tax revenues are used to buy coverage for the poor. With the government's dollar at stake, it is implausible that it will not exercise some fiduciary oversight. Second, society does not make people bear the full cost of error, folly, or turpitude with respect to their health care decisions. If someone fails to buy coverage with their health insurance voucher and appears at an emergency room, society will probably not condemn the person to die on the steps of the hospital.

Single-payer enthusiasts, with their distaste for markets and their confidence in government, readily design regulatory bodies and administrative agencies to overcome these hurdles. Marketists, though, see government failure lurking behind every streetlight on Pennsylvania Avenue. For the most part, their proposals avoid questions of institutional design.

The administrative requirements of moving from a market-based design like the original managed-competition proposal to one that provided universal coverage within a market bedeviled the Clinton task force. The managed-competition proposal, the most elaborate of the marketist schemes, calls for a market maker to provide quality assurance, plan certification, and countervailing bargaining power. The problems of moving beyond the market, even a small distance, can be seen in the problems of redesigning the central market-making institution in this model, the Health Insurance Purchasing Cooperative (HIPC).[18]

The HIPC, modeled after a farmers' cooperative, would allow consumers to pool their purchasing power in the insurance market. In the original managed-competition proposals, which did not provide for universal coverage, the consumers who pooled their purchasing power would be large corporations that voluntarily joined forces to negotiate with producers. An HIPC might include only a limited number of corporations, and many independent HIPCs could exist in one area. The HIPC, like a farmers' cooperative, would be managed by its members. The government's role, in the original proposal, was limited to changing the tax treatment of health insurance.

A number of large employers, acting singly, have proceeded with managed-competition-style reforms. The largest long-running managed-competition experiment is the Minnesota public employees program, in place since 1988. The program includes about 140,000 employees of the state of Minnesota. After the state standardized benefit packages, set a uniform contribution level for all plans, and began to require quality assessment information, the share of employees enrolled in the lowest-cost plan doubled. Since then, growth in enrollment in low-cost plans has continued.

Other managed-competition experiments show similarly encouraging results, although for shorter periods. The largest plan—the California Public Employee Retirement System (CALPers), which has operated as a managed-competition plan since 1991—has experienced average cost inflation less than the national average since 1992. Xerox and Digital Equipment Corporation also found that employees showed much greater willingness to choose HMOs when they were financially rewarded for this choice (Health Care Task Force 1993).[19]

Despite the apparent success of these programs, they have not spread quickly to other sites. Firms may have found the organizational costs of establishing managed competition daunting. Where corporations have established managed-competition plans, they have mainly done so alone.[20] Groups of corporations do not seem to have been able to overcome free-rider problems and establish managed-competition programs without government support.

Joint-purchasing organizations, modeled on HIPCs, have now become part of many marketist reform proposals, especially for the small-group market. In these proposals, as in the universal-coverage version of managed competition, however, purchasing groups are no longer spontaneous and voluntary creations of independent corporations. Rather, these models put a government agency in the role of creating HIPCs, and a separate government body has responsibility for defining a standard benefit package.

Using a government agency to create these institutions, rather than relying on voluntary action, overcomes initial organizational problems. These quasi-governmental purchasing groups, however, raise questions of administrative accountability. A HIPC formed by the voluntary cooperation of a small number of large firms has stakeholders who can reasonably be expected to negotiate with providers, enforce standards, operate a risk adjustment system, and develop measures for quality assessment. A purchasing group that incorporates small, transient firms cannot be expected to generate such accountable leadership. Plans with mandatory purchasing groups must (and do) have a larger role for government than envisioned in the original managed-competition plans, not only in establishing the institution but in maintaining it (Zelman 1993).

Once it is organized, someone must actually operate the purchasing group. Purchasing groups could be operated by government regulatory agencies or by government-chartered independent agencies, perhaps elected directly by voters. Government operation of the purchasing group, though, revives the concerns that led marketists to dislike single-payer-style reforms.

Mandatory purchasing cooperatives require considerable departures from the managed-competition ideal, even without infusions of government funding and in the absence of special concerns about the potential failure of participating insurers.[21] Nonetheless, it is possible to imagine that such a system could operate with privately administered purchasing groups that periodically let contracts to managers to operate nonoverlapping HIPCs. Once given public funds to cover care for the poor and ensure continued coverage, however, privately operated HIPCs become subject to standards of political accountability. Privately administered purchasing groups may not adequately address public health concerns or maintain culturally appropriate services for poor, underserved areas. In the original managed-competition conception, private HIPCs had no role in performing these functions. If purchasing groups were government-established entities with a significant role in financing health care, the scope of their activities would be likely to expand, and it would become much more difficult to write contracts that encouraged private managers to balance these varied objectives.[22]

Medicalist and Marketist Solutions to the Resource Allocation Problem

The institutional structures proposed by medicalists and marketists must respond to the changing nature of health care in two important respects: raising money and spending money. The latter problem is one of allocating resources within the health care system, and it is in this respect that the medicalist single-payer model and the marketist competing-payer model are most divergent. The single-payer model uses centralized allocation. Explicit technology constraints, legislated fee schedules, special benefits for well-organized groups, and limited organizational innovation are predictable consequences of this method. By contrast, the multiple-payer model uses a decentralized process to make allocation decisions; independent actors respond to prices. Duplicative technology, lavish salaries for scarce talents, and organizations that periodically fail are predictable consequences of this allocation method.

The single-payer model works best when components of medical practice can be divorced from one another and patterns of practice are stable. When only hospitals have the facilities to treat certain conditions and only doctors have the capacity to treat other ones, paying hospitals and doctors can be treated as (relatively) discrete issues. Allocation may not meet ideal market standards—a few favored doctors may have queues for their services (rather than charging higher prices and working more hours as they might in a market system), but the allocation problems will not be severe. Queues can even solve aspects of the allocation problem in the single-payer system. By observing queues, the payer can recognize a shortage and make corrections. Studies of waiting lines or rationing decisions in countries with waiting lines generally find that these lines correspond quite well to measures of medical need among waiting patients (GAO 1992b).

Centralized allocation systems perform less well when called upon to respond to rapidly changing situations, especially where many alternative choices exist. Consider the case of a condition previously treated in hospitals that can now be treated in an outpatient facility. In a single-payer system, the payer controls the mix of services by choosing of the number of surgical units to allocate to this condition. To make this choice rationally, the payer must know the prevalence of the condition and the relative cost-effectiveness of treating it in or out of hospital and in different kinds of cases. If beds are scarce, even costly outpatient treatment might be preferred to inpatient care. If beds abound, out-patient treatment may be a second choice. If the payer selects too small or too large a number of surgical units, costs will be higher than necessary. Finally, the payer must decide whether to expand or contract the overall health care budget in response to the innovation.

If such treatment innovations occur only sporadically, the regulator can do a reasonable job of making these decisions. More often, regulators will fall behind the pace of innovation. The process of recalibrating the system takes too long to merit changes for every minor innovation. Instead, regulators are likely to wait until innovations accumulate and then overhaul the system completely.

In the multiple-payer case, each hospital or pharmaceutical company offers its product (a hospital bed, outpatient facility, or drug) at a price it selects. Individual physicians and patients may then decide which course of treatment is most cost-effective for them. The allocations are made locally by hospitals and facilities on the basis of the information available to them. Some facilities may make the wrong choices and build too much capacity or fail to respond to an innovation. But other facilities, sensing an opportunity to profit, will likely step in to fill the gap. Change occurs continuously, and while allocations may be off-kilter for a time, adjustments will occur quickly.

As health care moves away from the simple distinctions between doctors and hospitals, and between drugs and surgery, and as our traditional understanding of medical need broadens to encompass social and personal characteristics, the benefits of rapid responses to changing technologies are likely to become more important. In this respect, the single-payer model fails the test of a successful health system: its institutional structures cannot respond quickly and flexibly to rapid change.

Medicalist and Marketist Solutions to the Financing Problem

In contrast to the sharp conflict over the allocation of resources, the medicalist and marketist models differ little in their approaches to raising money. Medicalists and marketists alike believe that the bulk of the funds for paying the cost of health care for the uninsured should be raised from general taxes designed, as a matter of tax policy, to balance the need to raise funds for redistribution against the negative effects of higher taxes on the taxpayers' willingness to work.

Differences between medicalists and marketists manifest themselves mainly with respect to out-of-pocket costs. Not surprisingly, given their tendency to deemphasize the effects of both personal behavior and the uncertainties of medical care on health outcomes, medicalists see no reason to make patients bear any costs and would eliminate individual payments altogether. Marketists, who accentuate the importance of human conduct both in becoming ill and in choosing services, would make individuals responsible for at least part of the costs of their own care.

Most plans that propose universal coverage though, whether medicalist or marketist, tend to ignore the effects of patient and provider behavior on the costs of the basic plan (or the amount of the tax credit). In a perfectly competitive market, the problem of average costs can safely be ignored. As long as consumers and providers face the marginal cost of their decisions (relative to locally available alternatives), they will minimize the total cost of producing and distributing goods and services. Approaches to health care reform that rely heavily on markets argue that much of the need for health planning and direct regulatory control of the supply side can be avoided by making consumers more cost conscious at the margin. Reliance on markets avoids the problems of government failure described in my discussion of the single-payer plan.

In the health care market, with its soup of public and private interests, and even in the more market-oriented version envisioned by marketist reformers, it is hard to be sanguine that the power of the pocketbook at the margin will defeat self-interested lobbies. Cost consciousness may ensure that consumers will seek out less expensive forms of care. Even informed, cost-conscious consumers, though, may not succeed in generating the political pressure to counter health care lobbies that impede price competition among physicians or keep inefficient hospitals going. Nor can intermediate service purchasers, such as insurers, necessarily counter these lobbies. Insurers as a group cannot expect to sell many more policies if they combine to lobby against regulations that increase health care prices. Under universal coverage with standard benefit packages, insurers' incentives for countervailing action may disappear altogether.[23]

Given the diverse interests of consumers and the concentrated benefits to producers of working together, it may be unrealistic to hope that consumer interests can counter producer interests at the political level simply by providing incentives at the margin. The problem can be seen by looking at the incentive effects of the financing scheme most favored by economic commentators.

Financing Health Care and Containing Costs

From an optimal tax perspective, many analysts believe that the ideal way to finance health care would be through a national value-added tax, or VAT. A national VAT could be designed to pay only for the cost of the lowest-priced plan in each region, the cost of a catastrophic-coverage plan in the area, or the cost of a health insurance voucher for local coverage, thus enabling everyone to afford some health coverage. Consumers would then pay all marginal costs associated with their plan choice. Indeed, the VAT was the first financing approach considered by the Clinton administration, although it was quickly rejected on political grounds.

Under a national VAT though, differences in the cost of care from region to region would be ignored. Regions would not be rewarded for bringing down the cost of their health care system as a whole, or penalized for raising average costs. The uncoupling of the VAT from regional health care costs means that the VAT rate could not be used as a focus of consumer concern that would counter provider lobbies. Indeed, rational consumers would prefer to drive up the cost of the lowest-cost plan in their region. The effect on their own VAT payments from an increase in local health costs would be trivially small, while the benefits of better hospitals and richer providers would accrue entirely to them. Under a VAT, local consumer pressure, not just provider pressure, would work against keeping costs down.

A national VAT combined with locally priced vouchers could set off a spiral of increasing health costs. On one hand, while all consumers would be better off if no states passed cost-increasing regulations, each state's residents would prefer for their own state to provide as many services as possible. On the other hand, setting a fixed national voucher level would make it impossible for poorer residents of high-cost states to obtain the care guaranteed in the basic benefit package.

The incentive effects of a national VAT illustrate the complexity of the connections between raising and disbursing health care revenues. A VAT that paid only for the price of the lowest-cost plan would leave people with appropriate incentives at the margin, but not at the average. Even without the strong connection between individual behavior and health costs posited by marketists, local tendencies toward increasing costs would erode cost containment in a fully VAT-based system. By failing to tie together revenues and expenditures, the fully VAT-based system would make enormous demands on the coercive global budgeting system to perform this cost-control function, and at the same time would gnaw away at the political will needed to support binding budgets.

The problems of a national VAT for funding health care occur because local patterns of medical care and local endowments of health care capital have such a significant influence on total health care costs. Locally based financing, through local payroll taxes or employer mandates, is much less desirable from the perspective of optimal tax policy. Employment-based financing distorts labor market decisions and hurts exporters. Local financing may also be undesirable from a health policy perspective. Without national oversight, states may compete in a race to the bottom, providing ever stingier benefits to their poor populations. If financing rates are allowed to vary from region to region, though, a local tax base may be more effective than a VAT in controlling health spending.

Transparent, local taxes for health care provide benchmarks that give incentives for cost containment. National taxes do not. In the United States, the dangers of national taxes can be seen most clearly in the case of the Medicare program. The Medicare tax raises revenues from one group (current workers) to pay for services to a different group (the elderly). Current workers and the elderly do not present a united front against providers. Medicare taxes do not vary across the country, so local decision making is insulated from its effects on Medicare costs. Finally, lawmakers have explicitly avoided making the Medicare tax rate a focus for cost containment efforts. Recent increases in Medicare payroll taxes have taken the less-than-transparent form of increases in the income cap.

Financing Health Care When Costs Rise

A system for financing health care should be structured to provide incentives for cost containment. At the same time, the system should generate enough revenue to cover the costs of the health program. In the medicalist structure, that means generating enough tax revenue to pay for the cost of health care for everyone. In the marketist model, it means generating enough revenue to provide health benefits to those who cannot afford to buy them.

In the medicalist model, the government takes an active role in deciding how much health care people should get. If the government believes taxes are too high, it can simply decide to reduce the amount it spends on health care. From a marketist perspective, though, this decision can lead to a reduction in health spending below the level that would make people best off. Arguably, the strict controls on health spending in Canada are an example of this situation. Many Canadians would be better off if they were permitted to divert some money from buying autos and VCRs to buying more rapid treatment and longer doctor visits. But medicalists willingly sacrifice consumer autonomy for egalitarianism. Financing care for the poor when costs rise need not be a problem in this model because costs need not rise.

Marketists assert that consumers should choose how much to spend on health care. As I noted in the previous section, even without rising costs, raising health care expenditures through broad-based taxes creates incentives to raise local spending. But no broad-based tax, whether local, regional, or national, will provide a stream of revenues that keeps pace with rising health costs. Neither federal Medicare taxes nor state Medicaid taxes have done so in the past. Instead, rising health expenditures will mean that without further action, tax revenues will not cover the costs of distributing an increasingly costly minimum package to the poor. The experiences of Medicare and Medicaid suggest that the government will try to reconcile the balance between revenues and costs by regulating the system further—for example, by reducing payments to the providers in the lowest-cost plans.

The marketist model lacks the internal consistency of the medicalist model, with its relentless emphasis on equality. Marketists built their plans to address problems in the operation of the health care market. As long as their models address these problems—the concerns of consumers who can afford their own care—the model remains internally consistent. But wherever redistributional concerns are grafted onto the marketist model, problems emerge. Providing health insurance to those in ill health requires the designing of standard benefit packages, a significant departure from the market. Improving access to health insurance for disadvantaged purchasers requires the government to establish and operate health insurance purchasing organizations. As creations of the political process, these organizations will have to respond to provider, consumer, and community concerns, again subverting the free market. Finally, financing health care for the poor through broad-based taxes while costs are allowed to grow freely is likely to bring further regulation to the system. The government's role in providing care for the poor may undermine the possibility that market competition will be permitted to lead to efficiency.

The institutional structure of the marketist model draws its strength from its single-minded responsiveness to the flow of dollars. That fixation is what permits the unregulated market to identify and exploit opportunities rapidly in an ever changing health care system. But for this very reason, the unfettered market cannot redistribute health care resources to those without dollars.

The medicalist structure divorces everyday decisions from dollars. Instead, it uses the political process to make decisions about the overall level of spending and the extent of redistribution. This attention to political concerns makes the medicalist structure a good way to redistribute resources, but a weaker means for responding to changing technologies, diverse organizational forms, and heterogeneous consumer preferences.

7 ///

Making Health Policy:
The Clinton Plan

Both medicalist and marketist models are undermined because they do not attend to the consequences of rapidly changing health care technologies. Furthermore, attempts to combine the dynamism of the market model with the benevolence of the medicalist model are likely to stumble. Regulatory constraints diminish the power of the unfettered market as a resource allocation device. Allowing costs to grow freely is incompatible with guaranteeing adequate care to the poor.

The experience of the Clinton administration illustrates many of the difficulties of designing a compromise between medicalists and marketists. Although the president's plan sought to use the market to allocate resources, it had to engage the political process to redistribute funds. The desire to achieve universal coverage opened the proposal to the importuning of special interests and required it to build institutional structures that would safeguard public money. The result was a plan too costly and too regulatory to sustain a market.

The Clinton administration's experience also highlights the importance of a new force, neither medicalist nor marketist, that is increasingly shaping health care policy: the imperative to control government health spending to deal with the federal deficit. While both marketists and medicalists participated in developing the Clinton plan and engaged in heated debates over health policy, their principled arguments

186

against regulation or in favor of more generous coverage for the poor were inevitably trumped by the mere mention of the federal deficit. The same compulsion to control the deficit quieted the ideological fervor of the 104th Congress's attempt to remake the Medicare program into a more marketist structure.

The linkage between health programs and growing government deficits exists precisely because neither type of institutional structure accommodates the dynamic nature of health care. The state of the federal budget when the Clinton administration took office simply gave immediate exposure to problems that would otherwise have become manifest with the passage of time.

President Clinton and Health Care

President Clinton's health plan was never grounded in any particular philosophy of health care. As a presidential candidate, Bill Clinton embarked on his campaign without any health care plan at all. Nebraska Senator Bob Kerrey, alone among Democrats in the 1992 primary elections, made universal health care a major campaign plank. Kerrey took a principled stance and proposed a single-payer plan along the lines of the Canadian system. Despite gaining the support of many health reform advocates, he finished no better than third in seven of the eight primaries he entered, and he withdrew from the campaign in March of 1992. As Clinton's support coalesced, his campaign team recognized that health reform could be a valuable tool in the campaign against George Bush. Health reform oriented toward secure universal coverage and cost containment could be a way of encouraging the middle class to believe that government could work for them.

Clinton's team initially adopted a pay-or-play health plan, the universal-coverage-oriented package put forward by Michael Dukakis in his 1988 presidential campaign. Pay-or-play plans require employers to purchase coverage for their employees or else pay a flat payroll tax for coverage through a public plan. Although marketists argue that such reforms would inevitably evolve into a government-run health system, the pay-or-play design itself makes relatively few institutional or ideological demands. The payroll tax element of the plan, however, makes it vulnerable to political attack. Within a few weeks of Clinton's advocacy of pay-or-play, the Congressional Republican Joint Economic Committee had estimates of the potential job losses associated with its payroll tax and the vast new public insurance program it would create. Job losses and big new public programs did not fit Clinton's image as a New Democrat.

By August 1992 Clinton had embraced a new plan based on a widely praised design developed in California that combined explicit cost control with a managed-competition framework, a compromise between markets and bureaucracies (Starr 1994). Although the California plan contained explicit payroll taxes and cost controls, the concept of mixing the old ideas of universal coverage and budget caps with the private-public partnerships, efficiency-enhancing incentives, consumer choice, and quality control of managed competition sounded quintessentially "New Democratic."

President Clinton's two stated objectives in undertaking health care reform were to cover the uninsured and to reduce the cost of care as a share of GDP and in the federal budget. Managed competition is not a plan for extending coverage or for directly reducing the cost of health care, although it might increase the efficiency of the health care system. It would directly address the federal budget by limiting the tax subsidy for the purchase of health insurance, but it had no implications for Medicare or Medicaid. Given his two objectives, it seems almost perverse that the president chose as a basis for his reform a plan that emphasized neither. Managed competition, a plan that called on the government to improve the functioning of the market, fit more closely with the administration's basic approach to public intervention in the private sector than with its health care concerns. Rather than confronting the private sector directly, as the single-payer plan would have, managed competition acknowledged the supremacy of the market, while providing a role for able public servants to improve its functioning.

Managed competition proved a rickety chassis on which to construct a plan that met the president's policy goals. Managed competition is a marketist-oriented plan, but the president's objectives—equitable universal coverage and guaranteed cost containment—fit more readily into a medicalist framework. Developing a managed-competition-based plan that would incorporate universal coverage and guarantee (rather than simply encourage) cost containment would require a fundamental reformulation of the original scheme. From the beginning, then, the plan would require a compromise between the president's goals and his policy model.

The President's Plan

As I noted in Chapter 1, the Clinton plan was designed to produce "competition under a budget." In the discussion that follows, I focus on a number of key components of the Clinton administration's plan to illustrate the points made in previous chapters. To put these components in context, I begin with a brief description of the final Clinton plan.

President Clinton's plan was built around five basic elements (see figure 7.1). First and foremost, the plan relied on a newly devised institution called a "regional health alliance." In each region of the country, the health alliance, a government-created purchasing organization, would organize and regulate the regional health insurance market. Second, health insurers and managed-care plans that conformed to certain quality and regulatory standards could sell their products through the health alliance at a price they themselves determined. All health plans would have to cover the same (comprehensive) services and adhere to government-established deductible and copayment levels. Third, em-

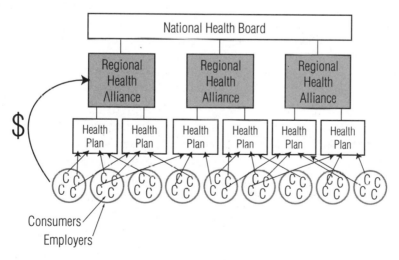

Figure 7.1 Organizational structure of the Clinton health reform plan

ployers would have to make premium payments to the alliance in their region, in amounts equal to 80 percent of the average cost of health plans offered in that alliance, on behalf of each of their employees. Premium payments for employers of low-wage workers would be capped, with the difference made up through federal subsidies.

Fourth, as in other managed-competition plans, consumers would make the decisions that drove the system, choosing among the array of health plans offered in the alliance. A consumer who chose a plan with average costs would pay 20 percent of the cost of that plan. Because the employer's contribution would be fixed at 80 percent of the average, a consumer who chose a less costly plan than average would pay less than 20 percent of the cost of that plan, and a consumer who chose a more costly plan than average would pay more than 20 percent of the cost. This pricing structure was intended to give consumers incentives to make decisions about health plans that took cost into account. By making price an important element of consumer decisions, this structure was intended to give health plan operators an incentive to keep costs down.

The alliance structure of the Clinton plan, the flat-contribution rule, the role of health plans, and the incentives provided to consumers and health plans were drawn almost directly from the marketist managed-competition plan. The fifth element of the structure, the role of the national government, however, introduced an element from the medicalist single-payer plan. The national government would determine the rate at which alliance premiums could rise. Since health plans would have government-established copayment and deductible levels and would cover a comprehensive array of benefits, and since, under the plan, doctors, hospitals, and other health providers could not charge patients extra for their services, the cap on premium growth would translate into a cap on most of national health spending. The cap formed the budget under which competition would operate.[1]

Much of the basic structure of this plan had been developed by the Clinton transition team before the administration came to Washington. The policy process in Washington responded to political, administrative, and financial pressures in moving from a theoretical outline to fully developed legislation. These responses demonstrate how most of the forces that shape health policy move toward increasing the regulatory component of any reform.

Resource Allocation through the Political Process: The Role of Special Interests

Although pollsters had trumpeted the public's interest in reform of the health care system, it quickly became apparent to those working on the plan that health reform could not realistically offer much to the American middle class. Most middle-class people already had insurance; they paid for it only indirectly (through their employers) and were unaware of its costs; and they were satisfied with the quality of their care. While the middle class might be sympathetic to health reform, they were unlikely to mount a campaign in its favor or to confront the lobby groups who would undoubtedly mass against it. Security of coverage was a genuine concern, but for most of the middle class loss of coverage was a distant risk, not an everyday problem. The uninsured, who would be served by reform of the system, had little political clout and were too preoccupied with the demands of their daily existence to mount a credible campaign for reform. The attempt to build a marketist-oriented reform hit an immediate stumbling block. The administration needed vociferous supporters for its plan, so it had to be receptive to the admonitions of powerful interest groups. These groups stripped the plan of some important cost-containment features and vastly expanded its scope.

Three groups were potential advocates for health reform: labor unions, big business, and the elderly. While ideologically miles apart, the self-interests of labor unions and many older big businesses were aligned. Both groups wanted the government to shift the costs of health care from employment to a tax-based system, away from them and toward taxpayers in general.

The need to generate union and business support for the health plan scotched the most important element of marketist proposals: reforming the tax subsidy for employer-provided health insurance. The health insurance tax subsidy is distortionary, regressive, and costly. It provides tax breaks to upper-income taxpayers and rewards those who choose costly and inefficient health plans. The principal beneficiaries of the favorable tax treatment given to health insurance, however, are well-insured and vocal union members and upper-middle-income taxpayers (Glied 1994). Union opposition to the tax cap was so strong that even a stripped-down cap would only have been phased in over time under the Clinton plan.

Beyond its various benefits as a health policy measure, reforming the tax treatment of health insurance would have had short-term and long-term revenue benefits. A tax cap immediately generates savings (additional federal revenues) and protects the federal budget from increases in private health costs. A midlevel tax cap would have saved as much as $19 billion in federal revenue each year (CBO 1994a).

Including a tax cap in a health reform proposal might have made it unsalable to unions and business groups. Not including it, though, was hardly a reason for them to offer their enthusiastic support. In an attempt to improve the plan's prospects, the administration eventually added a direct payoff to business supporters. It promised to take over the costs of health benefit plans for retirees over fifty-five. Paying early-retiree health benefits with taxpayer money made no fiscal or health policy sense; it did not pull the plan toward either the medicalist or the marketist model; it was simply a political payoff—to the tune of about $100 million a year, valued only by the subset of businesses that had many retirees (OMB 1994).

The most important health lobby group, especially after the Catastrophic Act debacle, are the elderly. Upon Clinton's election elderly Americans bombarded the White House with letters demanding assistance with prescription drug costs and long-term care. Both issues had real policy salience. Medicare does not pay for the cost of prescription drugs or for long-term care, and many poor elderly Americans were hard pressed to afford these expenses. But while these problems obviously begged for solutions, it was less clear that the solutions should be incorporated in the overall health reform plan. The administration's health policy plans did not contemplate a reformulation of the Medicare program. Any new benefits offered to the elderly would operate independent of the managed-competition system being designed for people under sixty-five. Although new programs for the elderly might be warranted on health policy grounds, political considerations motivated the decision to include them in the president's plan.

Politics, rather than policy, explains the design of the programs for the elderly that were incorporated in the president's plan. Advocacy groups for senior citizens, funded mainly by middle- and upper-income older people, wanted any new programs to provide universal coverage, not coverage based on income. A non-means-tested, pay-as-you-go, universal long-term-care program would have been immensely costly, especially once the baby boomers begin retiring twenty years from now. The final plan's much more restricted proposal, a capped, non-means-tested program, met a political test, but it failed miserably as policy. States would be given limited block grants to provide more home care services to the elderly and disabled, but they would not be permitted to allocate these funds on the basis of financial need. The prescription drug proposal would have extended existing Medicare coverage to these medications, providing new subsidized benefits to all elderly Americans, including those who already owned private policies covering prescription drugs. A generous prescription drug policy would have led the elderly to spend about $10 billion more on drugs than they were already, but because costs previously covered by private insurance and out-of-pocket spending would now be covered by Medicare, the benefit would cost the U.S. Treasury $25.4 billion.

There was nothing unusual or heinous about the Clinton administration's desire to woo unions, big business, and the elderly. Just as theory predicts, however, the pursuit of political support from these groups substantially increased the cost of its health plan. That increase in cost made the financing of the plan more precarious. The extra benefits also made the structure, already hard to make out, even more obscure. The benefits provided to the elderly alone added more than 100 pages to the text of the Health Security Act.

Plan supporters demanded costly special benefits, but likely opponents, too, could demand, and receive, favors in return for turning down the volume of their opposition. Physician groups complained that the plan gave managed-care organizations too much control over the profession. The administration responded by requiring that regional health alliances include as many fee-for-service plans as entered the market, and that every HMO plan have a point-of-service option allowing patients to choose any provider they wanted (at a defined additional cost). Insurers complained that regional health alliances would be able to exclude costly plans arbitrarily. The administration responded by reducing the power of the health alliances. People with low coinsurance and low-deductible plans complained that they would be forced to take on higher coinsurance and deductibles under the plan. The administration responded by allowing employers to reimburse employees for coinsurance and deductible costs without paying taxes on the additional compensation.

The administration's attempt to bolster the market with a light superstructure of regulation opened a Pandora's box of special favors. The specter of regulation to contain costs and extend coverage created an opportunity for regulation to promote special interests.

Overseeing Public Funds: Centralization and Decentralization

Any reform proposal that promised to cover the uninsured would require taking money from some Americans and giving it to others. Like any redistributive program, the health care plan had to include enough oversight to ensure that resources would not be squandered or misappropriated. Combining the promise of universal coverage with a goal of cost containment raised the stakes of that oversight function. The administrators of the Clinton health plan would have to watch their program's money carefully. While public resources are most easily supervised in a highly centralized, regulated system, however, such a system would be inimical to the operation of a free market. The plan had to trade off the policy and, often, political benefits of a decentralized system against the need to control the flow of resources. These tensions played themselves out in debates between the health policy academics and the federal civil servants who participated in President Clinton's health care task force.

The Health Care Task Force

The health care task force has been the subject of extraordinary misconceptions. It generated enormous controversy, even a lawsuit. For all its notoriety, however, the health care task force depended almost entirely on the preexisting government bureaucracy for its expertise. Of the 500 members of the Clinton health care task force, the vast majority were federal civil servants (BNA 1993).[2] Rules against conflicts of interest meant that no insurance company executives, hospital executives, or representatives of HMOs could join the task force. Very few of the people on the task force had any experience in the operation of the private insurance industry. No successful insurance company executive was willing to give up his job to participate in the task force. Instead, the federal bureaucrats were joined by a few consultants, insurance regulators, and academics.

In the development of the president's plan, the federal employees were persistent advocates for a more tightly controlled system. Since bureaucrats will be called to account for program failures, they understandably prefer a program they can easily monitor and regulate. Furthermore, in a world of five-year budget projections, bureaucrats sensibly focus on the effects of a program in the near term.[3]

In the Clinton task force, most civil servants came from the Department of Health and Human Services. Among its other functions, the department collects all data on national and state health costs, employs most of the health analysts in Washington, and produces cost projections for all federal health programs.[4]

This wealth of information means that the Department of Health and Human Services bureaucracy is indispensable to federal health reform efforts. The composition of the task force was not a sign of bias in the Clinton administration's plan. It simply reflected the reality of the expertise available in Washington. The same people who worked on the Clinton task force had spent the previous 12 years working on health policy under Republican administrations.[5]

The bureaucracy's agenda, which emphasizes the importance of rules, data, and regulatory oversight, enjoys elevated status in a world of limited public funds. The strains between the bureaucrats' emphasis on the need for control and the marketists' desire for decentralization is illustrated by the debates that occurred over two important components of the Clinton plan: the role of the states and the mechanism for raising revenues.

Federal or State Control?

Possible models of national health reform in the United States ranged from a Canadian-style system, with a few basic principles, a federal block grant, and free rein to the states, to a fully developed centralized system that would be implemented and managed by the federal government (such as extending Medicare to cover the whole population). Options between these poles included providing a fallback model for states that could not or would not choose an acceptable plan, imposing a standard plan and requiring states to obtain waivers for alternate ones, and designing multiple options from which states could choose (Kronick 1993; Mashaw 1993).

Initially, the president's plan envisioned considerable state flexibility, perhaps reflecting Clinton's own background as a governor. Historically, both the insurance industry and the practice of medicine have been regulated at the state level. The diversity in state regulations, for example, contributed to faster development of HMOs in some states than in others. States, too, had moved faster and in more innovative ways to reform health care than had the federal government. Hawaii, acting alone, was the only place in the country to have near-universal coverage; California and Minnesota both created forms of managed competition for public employees; and some states seriously considered single-payer legislation.

Advocates of state flexibility expounded the traditional federalist view of states as laboratories of democracy and pointed to existing reform experiments in various states as evidence of states' ability to design health programs tailored to their specific needs. These policymakers tended to express uncertainty about what the correct design of reform should be and saw state experimentation as a way of converging on the best plan. State-flexibility advocates also noted that state regulators had far more experience with the regulation of private insurance markets than did federal regulators and would be better able to design managed-competition-style reforms.

The president's tendency toward state flexibility, however, ran counter to the need to maintain control over the system. Advocates of central government control argued that many states had neither the political will nor the capacity to design and run their own programs. These planners emphasized the inability of the federal government to guarantee adequate treatment for the poor and to regulate costs under a more flexible system. They particularly feared misuse of federal funds and gaming of the federal funding mechanism by states. Large employers, with operations in many states, were concerned about coping with 50 different sets of regulations.

The strongest advocates of a federal program were federal bureaucrats. While many bureaucrats may have preferred a federal program because it would entrench the power of the federal bureaucracy and enhance the status of their own positions, they had good reason for fearing a state-run program, given their experience with Medicaid. After monitoring the Medicaid programs for more than 30 years, federal Medicaid bureaucrats do not trust the states with either financial responsibility or program responsibility (GAO 1993a). While some states have run exemplary Medicaid programs, others fulfill only the bare letter of their obligations. All states make every effort to extract as many dollars as possible from the federal government. In the late 1980s, they were notoriously successful: federal Medicaid spending was driven up at annual rates of 35 percent through innovative schemes like the tax-and-donation programs in which hospitals paid special state taxes and were compensated by being granted an increase in their Medicaid rates, which, in turn, were partially paid by the federal government.

Federal bureaucrats, burned by past experience, insisted that if states were going to be given responsibility for running their health plans, they should be required to share responsibility for the costs incurred. If the president's plan was going to contain national—federal—health expenditures, they argued, the federal government should increase its contribution to state spending only in accordance with a strictly limited update formula. Any excess spending would have to be raised entirely by the states.

Under the Medicaid program, states had been required to pay 20 to 50 percent of any increase in program expenditures. During the 1980s, as the federal government expanded coverage in the Medicaid program, states found themselves left with health care bills for services they had not legislated. In light of this experience, governors, like the federal bureaucracy, had legitimate concerns about a system in which the federal government made broad coverage decisions, defined a basic benefit package, and decided how quickly costs could rise, while leaving states with full responsibility for cost overruns.

The governors' concerns heightened as the president's global-budget mechanism became tighter. Allowing the states to make up the cost of overruns would protect the federal budget, but, said cost estimators, it would not check the growth in national health spending. To meet the president's promise of health cost containment, states that exceeded their budgets would not only have to make up the excess cost, they would also have to pay explicit penalties for breaking the federally established budget. Faced with the prospect of significant and punitive health costs, the governors balked.

State flexibility is clearly incompatible with a stringent global budget that limits national health spending. In Canada the federal government does not limit national spending. Nonetheless, as the Canadian federal government has reduced its contribution to provincial plans, provinces have begun to ignore federal regulatory requirements. Some provinces have considered allowing physicians to balance-bill patients above the fee schedule or to open private clinics, counter to federal regulations. In effect, the federal government has lost leverage over the provinces.

But it is not clear that state flexibility in a U.S. health reform plan could have survived even a softer budget. The federal-state division of responsibility for the Medicaid program has led to mistrust and conflict. State governors do not relish the prospect of putting their funds at the mercy of federal policymakers; federal bureaucrats, often opposed by lawmakers sympathetic to the states' travails, have failed to stem the deliberate hemorrhaging of federal Medicaid funding. In this atmosphere, decisions about the appropriate compass of federal and state action in health care were made on the basis of fiscal realities rather than on underlying health reform or federalist theory. Although President Clinton was sympathetic to the idea of state flexibility, it was not a critical element of his plan. Faced with the choice between potential cost overruns and a federal system, the administration chose to keep the reins tight and in Washington.

Financing Health Care

Within the administration it quickly became clear that the role of the task force was to design the best possible health plan. The cabinet, with its regular staff, would figure out how to pay for it. This arrangement implicitly suggested that the structure of the plan would in no way depend on its financing, an approach that is typical of both marketist and medicalist proposals, as I noted in Chapter 6. Health policy would influence only the design of the plan; politics would determine how it was financed.

Three options were considered to finance the health plan. Initially, the administration contemplated introducing a new value-added tax (a form of sales tax) to finance the full costs of national health expenditures other than copayments and deductibles and the marginal costs of higher-cost health plans.

The VAT was rejected because of the high tax rate that would be needed in order to fund all of health care except out-of-pocket payments. To do that in 1996 would have meant raising about $900 billion from a consumption base of $3.6 trillion ($1.9 trillion excluding food, medical care, and other necessities; CBO 1994b). Tax payments made through the VAT would reduce labor income and corporate revenues and hence the taxes on those items. This "tax offset" implied that to make the treasury whole and raise the money for health care would require a VAT rate in the teens.[6]

Focus groups, unsurprisingly, showed a notable lack of enthusiasm for a VAT rate of 9 to 18 percent. White House scuttlebutt hinted that elderly members of the focus groups were particularly incensed. They complained that they had already paid for their health care through Medicare payroll taxes while they were younger and considered it unfair to be required to pay again through sales taxes. In light of this very negative response, the VAT was summarily dismissed from consideration.

An employer mandate was the most obvious way of funding universal coverage in an employment-based system. More than 60 percent of all Americans under sixty-five already purchase health insurance through their employers; the employer mandate would simply extend this pattern to the others. Low-income workers, who could not afford to pay the mandated cost, would be subsidized. The apparent simplicity of extending the current system through an employer mandate, though, breaks down on closer inspection.

Under a voluntary system, workers accept and reject health insurance according to their own needs. If they overpay for coverage, they can blame only themselves. In 1987, for example, 28 percent of workers in dual-earner households bought double coverage—both spouses bought family insurance (Schur and Taylor 1991). In a compulsory system, every cranny in the byzantine structure of the American labor market requires a separate rule. Workers who are employed in multiple jobs, who work part-time, or who work part-year pose particular challenges. Must an employer cover a moonlighting worker who is already covered through his or her daytime employer? Should there be a proportional mandate for part-time workers? Should seasonal workers be expected to pay for all their health insurance during their period of employment? How do noncustodial divorced parents meet their insurance obligations? Subsidizing low-wage workers requires an additional set of rules and an additional pot of money to fund the subsidies.

The complexity of administering the employer mandate, more than any labor market or health policy concern, encouraged the administration to consider using a payroll tax to fund the health care program. A payroll tax is simpler than an employer mandate because it papers over the complexities underlying a mandate system and requires no special subsidies. In accomplishing this, the payroll tax generates significant redistributions, not only across incomes but across types of families and employment relationships.

The extent of redistribution under a payroll tax depends on its form. Using a simple flat-rate tax means that high-income workers will pay far more for health care than the cost of their premiums and low-income workers will pay far less. From a political perspective, this kind of redistribution is both a benefit and a curse: a benefit because subsidies to the poor are hidden within the overall payroll tax (or, as the administration preferred to call it, the "wage-based premium") and a curse because it could turn both high-income taxpayers and high-paying industries against reform.[7]

An even more politically volatile distributional problem emerged because the administration had decided to levy the payroll tax through the states. Giving each state its own payroll tax rate had the political benefit of converting a federal tax increase into a state tax increase, and it also increased state accountability for cost containment in the program. Under a payroll tax, though, subsidies for the poor would be lumped into the financing of the overall program rather than paid through a separate federal revenue source. States with low average earnings and many poor people (such as Arkansas and Louisiana) would have been required to levy taxes much higher than those needed in richer states (such as Connecticut).

Administratively and economically, the payroll tax was simpler and less distortionary than the employer mandate (with subsidies). But compared to the status quo, the payroll approach would have had too many losers: too many people would have paid much more than they were currently paying for health care. The employer mandate, despite its manifold flaws, had the virtue of leaving most already insured people more or less where they started.

Decisions about the VAT, the payroll tax, and the employer mandate were, for the most part, the focus of macroeconomic, labor market, and political concern. But decisions about financing had significant implications for the locus of control of health reform.

A VAT-based financing scheme would generate a highly centralized health care system. Alliances would have had to cover everyone—without any exemption for large corporations, since their employees, like everyone else, would be paying the VAT. The VAT, by its nature, would have been a national tax, eliminating any possible state role in the system. Virtually all the funding for the health care system would be disbursed by the U.S. Treasury, for which the VAT would be an enormous new responsibility. At $900 billion, revenue from the VAT would exceed that from the personal and corporate income tax. With all funding flowing in and out of Washington, the federal government would necessarily be directly responsible for any increases in health care costs, no matter where. If health care costs grew faster than overall consumption, the federal government would have had to raise the highly visible VAT rate or impose regulations to control costs.

A state-level payroll tax would have moved control to the state level. A payroll tax system could not permit large firms to opt out (or high-income workers in good health would leave the system, causing rates for those who remained to rise in a typical adverse-selection spiral). Under a state-levied payroll tax, the federal government would have found it much harder to impose constraints on the system. A system in which the states raised all the funds but the federal government made all the rules and exacted penalties for breaking them would be rather unstable. With states responsible for setting and adjusting payroll taxes, control over costs would be vested in state political decisions, not markets.

A pure employer mandate would have decentralized control over the health care system, leaving most decisions to markets. Firms and workers paying health care bills would have affected health care costs primarily as consumers. Large firms with highly paid workers could easily dispense with the health alliance system altogether. But an employer mandate, perhaps combined with individual subsidies, would have made it very difficult for the government to monitor the use of subsidy funds, maintain the equity of the system, and credibly promise to rein in total health care spending. If employees persuaded their employers to offer more generous health insurance at no cost to the government, it would have been very difficult to prohibit such coverage.

The president eventually selected a financing scheme that blended the employer mandate with the payroll tax. Firms would pay lump-sum mandated amounts, but payments could not exceed a nationally fixed percentage of (firmwide) payroll. This hybrid scheme meant that the extent of federal involvement (or, conversely, decentralization) in the plan depended on the relationship between health care costs and the cap rate. If very few employers fell under the cap, the plan could operate in a decentralized fashion. If most employers were capped, the plan would become dependent on funds raised in Washington and, almost certainly, more heavily regulated. In effect, if costs rose, the plan would move away from markets toward a more centralized structure.

Health Policy and the Federal Budget

The Clinton administration's first major obstacle upon reaching office was the budget deficit. The 1992 federal deficit stood at $290 billion. The president vowed to cut it in half—by $145 billion—within five years (Greenhouse 1992). The deficit affected the health plan immediately. In an effort to make deficit reduction easier, the administration considered a plan to tie health care reform to immediate budget reduction. Rather than waiting three months for the task force to complete its work, the president considered including health care savings in the budget speech he planned to make in February 1993.

Clearly, the administration could not hope to devise and budget an entire health plan in three weeks. Some advisers suggested instead that the president should use the budget speech to announce the immediate implementation of a short-term cost control strategy for health care. Savings from the short-term controls could be used to reduce the federal budget deficit. In addition to the potential budgetary savings, short-term cost containment might also encourage providers to negotiate seriously about the eventual direction of health reform, in an effort to remove the burden of controls.

Public Regulation, Private Savings:
The Debate over Short-Term Cost Containment

Although the possibility of such controls was first raised in relation to
the budget, short-term controls continued to be debated throughout
the existence of the health care task force. The internal debate over
short-term controls was particularly contentious because the form of
any short-term controls would almost certainly guide the implementation of the long-term strategy. If the short-term control strategy was
designed and put in place before the long-term one, it would likely
have more impact on the final design of health policy than would the
widely publicized managed-competition plan.

Three strategies for short-term cost containment were seriously considered: a freeze on all health care prices, imposition of Medicare rates
on the entire health system, and caps on insurance premiums. Richard
Nixon had ordered a freeze on health care prices during the wage-and-
price-control period of the 1970s. Health care prices had, indeed, sta-
bilized, only to skyrocket again when the freeze was lifted. Some conservatives liked the freeze because by its nature it could not continue
indefinitely and because it did not change the existing health care system. From a political perspective, however, a freeze initiated by the new
president would have looked hasty and frightening, and would have
reminded people of Nixon, a similarity that was viewed as a serious
liability (Priest 1993b).

The debate over the remaining two strategies, Medicare rate setting
and premium caps, masked a more profound debate over the direction
of health policy. Choosing rate setting would have meant moving health
reform toward the medicalist model and placing the federal Medicare
bureaucracy at the center of the health system. Premium caps, by contrast, would have entrenched insurance companies and generated an
inherently decentralized system. For true marketists, who disliked controls altogether, the premium-control option existed as a diversionary
tactic (Neuffer 1993). Many of those who appeared to favor premium
controls as an alternative to rate setting really preferred no controls at
all. The premium-control strategy allowed them to point out the difficulties of rate setting, the most realistic control strategy, without appearing to criticize the very idea of controls.

Under rate controls, all providers would have been required to implement Medicare-style rates developed through the Department of Health and Human Services. Prices to individual providers would have been controlled and insurers thus prevented from competing by signing up doctors at lower rates or directing all their business to specific hospitals. Only insurers who met stringent criteria would have been allowed to pay providers using capitation. Once the bureaucracy of rate setting was in place, insurers could not compete by forming networks of lower-cost providers or paying providers using incentives and would be relegated to their traditional role as payment conduits. Insurers, who were the basis of the managed-competition proposal, would have no further role to play; costs would be controlled by simply lowering prices. Furthermore, implementing rate setting would have been a significant exercise of government authority with respect to health care. It is unlikely that the political system or the health care system could manage two significant structural reforms—rate setting followed by managed competition—over a short period.

The case for premium controls was weak. Such controls had never been implemented anywhere and were sure to wreak havoc on the insurance industry, probably leading to temporary losses in insurance coverage for many people. From the perspective of some, though, a control strategy that depended on monitoring insurance premiums would cement the existence of private insurance in the new health system. Furthermore, premium controls would spur the implementation of health alliances, the structural basis of the long-term strategy. Without further institutional reform, premiums could not be monitored for long. Otherwise, insurers facing cost pressure would change the scope and nature of covered benefits as a means of avoiding controls.

Medicare rate setting meant accepting the policy prescription of the medicalist model. Premium controls were an intermediate step. Premium controls entrenched insurance companies, and so favored the market-oriented approach; but they also placed regulatory limits on health spending. Controls of any type were inimical to marketists. In the end there was no consensus about which strategy to adopt.

The search for short-term cost savings was ultimately abandoned because it became apparent that no system of short-term controls would have much impact on the budget deficit. As I indicated above, controlling costs is easiest in a highly centralized health care system—one where the regulators' money is on the line. The American health care system was (and continues to be) a relatively decentralized system. Most of the money in the system comes from outside the government. As a consequence, any short-term regulatory program would require massive intervention in private markets and would yield few budget savings. An absolute freeze on all health rates would have yielded less than $20 billion in savings in federal health programs over five years. In the private sector, short-term controls would have saved considerably more (some $50 billion to $70 billion), but Medicare and Medicaid rates were already virtually frozen. In order to use private health savings to balance the federal budget, the government would have had to "recapture"—Washington lingo for tax—private health care savings. Avoiding taxes was the principal reason for looking to health care savings in February in the first place.

Global Budgets: Federal-Deficit Reduction Transforms the Health Policy Debate

Once the capped employer-mandate financing arrangement described above was selected, the disjunction between public regulation and public-sector savings that had sunk short-term cost containment disappeared. Now regulation of the health care sector would not only meet policy goals of equity and cost containment: it would also have tangible effects on the federal budget. In a world of tight budgets, centralized financing greatly enhanced the appeal of regulation. The role of the federal deficit in health policy is well illustrated by the evolution of the Clinton plan's global budget.

President Clinton's design for health care reform called for managed competition under a global budget. Although managed competition had not been fully implemented on a large scale, there existed an extensive body of academic literature describing it, at least in terms of theory. A global budget for the entire health care system was a less well-developed concept, especially in conjunction with managed competition.[8]

Tacking a global budget onto managed competition solved important political problems. The president had stressed the importance of cutting the growth of health care spending and reducing the share of health care in the GDP, but many analysts were skeptical about the ability of managed competition to reduce spending growth. Underscoring this concern, Robert Reischauer, the director of the Congressional Budget Office, who would eventually be called upon to assess the financial impact of the plan, testified before Congress in February 1993 that he did not expect managed competition to achieve significant reductions in health spending (Reischauer 1993). The global budget would reassure skeptics—and the Congressional Budget Office—that the president's plan would, in fact, reduce health spending. The global budget would act as a backstop on managed competition.

A number of policy analysts have spoken and written in favor of the backstop (Aaron 1994; Starr 1994). But the perceived need for a backstop for a program as revolutionary as health reform is unsettling. The budget acts as a kind of redundant political engineering. Rather than waiting to see whether a new health system works well and modifying it after the fact if it does not, Congress would pass two different health plans at once. The budget-as-backstop strategy implicitly assumed that if a newly legislated system subsequently failed, the Congress and the president would find it very difficult to repair—or repeal—it.

The distressing charge of "political sclerosis" in U.S. health policy may be well founded. The long intervals between attempts at reform of the system over the past 60 years suggest that Congress can only rarely muster the energy for a serious pass at overhauling health care. The example of Medicare, which soon after its introduction was captured by potent interest groups highly resistant to change, suggests that health entitlements may be impossible to alter once in place. This resistance to change, though, raises real questions about the ability of the U.S. political system to operate a national health care program in a context of rapid technological change. In other countries with national health care systems, health care is a subject that receives frequent government attention, particularly in response to rising costs. If, as backstop proponents imply, American political institutions are not capable of modifying a system once it has been put in place, perhaps officials should be wary of implementing anything new.

If the global budget were simply a backstop for the managed-competition system, then setting budget levels would involve a determination of how much cost growth would be acceptable before shifting to an alternative strategy. The stringency of the global budget, then, would determine how much "managed competition" would be permitted in the health care system.

Medicalists preferred a comprehensive global budget. Restraining overall spending would limit inequities in the system by constraining the spending patterns of wealthier Americans. Federal bureaucrats favored a comprehensive, binding budget because it would encourage centralized monitoring and control over all health spending. Clearly, monitoring and control would be much simpler in a single-payer system in which all bills were paid centrally.

Marketists recognized that any binding global budget would undermine the incentives of managed competition (Roberts and Clyde 1993). This group lobbied for a generous budget that would give pure managed competition an opportunity to function and would simply measure costs and other data that could easily be collected within the managed-competition framework. They advocated for budget enforcement mechanisms that relied on the continued existence of competing insurers.[9]

While marketists and medicalists debated the principles behind a budget formula, the backstop model of the global budget fell by the wayside because of the need to prove that the health system could produce real savings overall, and especially in the federal budget. Any significant reduction in the rate of growth of health care in GDP would require a budget below the level of spending that analysts at the Congressional Budget Office and the Health Care Financing Administration predicted would emerge from an unfettered managed-competition system.

The regulators at the Health Care Financing Administration who ran the Medicare program promised that tightening the private-sector global budget would permit reductions in federal health spending. Normally, cutting public programs increases the risk that providers will turn away program beneficiaries. Medicare officials argued that under a system where all payers were equally constrained, cuts in public programs would have little impact on beneficiary access to services. In the context of a managed-competition reform, this argument was somewhat slim. Under managed competition, savings would presumably result from better management of service volume and new contractual arrangements between providers and payers, not from simple reductions in prices. Managed competition alone might reduce access for Medicare beneficiaries by pulling physicians into exclusive contracts with managed-care firms. In any case, the Clinton health plan envisioned that substantial reductions in provider fees (20 percent in real terms) were feasible if private health care costs were held within global caps (Kronick 1993).

The possibility of controlling Medicare spending by controlling private spending had been the main source of federal savings in the short-term cost containment plan. In the relatively centralized health system that would exist under the Clinton plan, large permanent rate reductions could be enforced, yielding substantially more savings than were available in the short-term plan. Furthermore, the global budget would credibly limit future liabilities from the new program, and it would also improve the federal balance sheet by reducing the cost of the federal tax expenditure associated with private health insurance premiums.

In the final plan, the global budget, translated into caps on spending in the public and private sectors, completed the financing of universal coverage and program expansions. The caps would balance program costs and revenues like closing the opposing blades of a pair of scissors. They would hold down the upper blade of the scissors, private insurance premiums and subsidy payments, preventing new federal costs from escalating. The cap would also raise paper savings in public programs, by holding the growth in these programs below projected rates.

This system generated a propitious relationship between the health plan and the federal deficit. The cap rate could be set to make the system self-financing, but it also could be set to raise money against the projected federal deficit. The cap rate in the final plan generated significant budget savings. It was set only slightly higher than the inflation rate—about half the current rate of growth in health spending. Although the final cap rate would have helped to balance the budget, it seems very unlikely that it would have permitted the operation of a managed-competition system. Among all the countries in the OECD, only one, Ireland, kept cost growth below the rate envisioned by the plan throughout the 1980s.

The decision to make the global budget immediately binding completely transformed the apparently marketist health plan into a highly regulatory medicalist plan. The strict enforcement provisions of the global-budget mechanism, rigid enough to satisfy the scrutiny of the

Congressional Budget Office, would have quickly moved control of the health system from regional health alliances to Washington regulators.

It would be a mistake to view the victory of the medicalist model as the consequence of deliberate plotting by federal regulators, the Congressional Budget Office, or medicalists. The budget agencies did their jobs with appropriate prudence, protecting the federal budget from overzealous reformers. Medicalists never liked the Clinton plan because it left insurance companies in place (even if their long-term survival seemed questionable) and decentralized funding through the employer mandate. The tight global budget certainly corresponded to the objectives of these groups, but its centrality in the plan was a result of neither the marketist nor the medicalist model of health care, but a crucial third force—the need to hold down federal health spending.

The Final Plan

Despite the efforts at building political support and engineering compromises, President Clinton's final health proposal, codified in the Health Security Act, combined elements of both marketist and medicalist proposals in a way that satisfied neither group. The plan had a managed-competition (marketist) infrastructure. Under the act, everyone not eligible for Medicare and not employed by a firm with more than 5,000 employees (or not a dependent of such an employee), would purchase a federally mandated, standardized insurance benefit package, usually from a private insurance company through a government-created "health alliance." Medicalists disliked the managed-competition structure of the plan, and its reliance on private insurers. They viewed private insurers and premiums as unnecessary and were particularly unhappy that the Clinton plan created yet another layer of bureaucracy between patient and doctor.

The plan also incorporated a medicalist regulatory structure through the global budget. The federal government would regulate the rate of increase in the weighted average premium of plans sold in the health alliances and prohibit billing in excess of established fee schedules. The budget was designed in terms of average health insurance premiums to avoid regulation of individual prices and permit some organizational flexibility (such as the development of integrated delivery systems).

Even under the best possible design, though, budgets and competition are an uneasy pairing. Binding global budgets must prohibit some people from buying more health care when they want it, and this subverts the individual preferences that are the basis of the market-oriented model. Marketists found these heavily regulatory elements of the plan extremely troublesome.

Yet the structure of the Health Security Act interwove elements from both models in a way that made it hard to disassemble. Marketists hated the premium controls, but without these limits the plan had no financing. If costs rose, all firms would fall under the payroll cap and Washington would become responsible for the full increment in health spending. Medicalists disliked the health alliances of competing insurers, but without them, a budget based on premium increases is not administratively feasible.

Even the groups that had been given special favors in the plan found it difficult to embrace. The elderly gained benefits, but lost considerable Medicare funding. Unions were spared the tax cap, but the standard benefit package offered in the plan was less generous than what they had already been receiving, making it a hard sell to workers. Big business saw overarching government interference in the health care system.

The president's reform proposal tried to chart a course for the future that would combine the conflicting visions of marketists and medicalists. It sought to exploit the strengths of the market in encouraging innovation while generating a more equal distribution of health care between the rich and the poor. Managed competition addressed the problems of bureaucracy-driven stagnation in health resource allocation that can occur in medicalist models when health care technologies change. The global budget addressed the problems of insufficient public funding that can occur in marketist models when health care costs rise. But rather than putting together the best of both worldviews, the Clinton plan was fundamentally flawed. Put simply, markets work only through prices, but global budgets regulate prices and limit the quantity of services that will be available. When health care changes as a result of the inevitable development of new and valued medical technology, the global budget becomes incompatible with managed competition.

The 1995 Attempt at Medicare Reform

President Clinton's health care reform proposal was resoundingly defeated. The 1994 congressional elections brought a Republican House and Senate to Washington, vocal partisans of free markets and less government. Health reform was not a priority for the 104th Congress; but reducing the federal deficit was part of its Republican members' "Contract with America." Health care spending through Medicare and Medicaid drove the federal deficit, forcing legislators to return to health policy.

In keeping with the Republican majority's antiregulatory philosophy, the Congress initially considered a thoroughly marketist reform of the heavily regulated, centralized Medicare program. Elderly Americans would be given vouchers and could go out into the market and buy the plans that pleased them. Competition among plans would keep costs down without further government action. This lofty vision quickly tumbled in a sequence familiar from the Clinton debate. An entirely unregulated market could not guarantee the amount of redistribution Americans wanted from the Medicare program. The government had to assure beneficiaries that they could continue to obtain the benefits Medicare had always promised. But if these benefits were to be maintained, the federal budget would continue to be at significant financial risk. Limiting that risk required imposing a substantial layer of regulation over the program. Once Congress recognized the magnitude of savings that could be achieved simply by cutting the rate of growth in Medicare, the lure of further regulation proved irresistible.

A pure voucher system would have required all Medicare beneficiaries to join private health plans (including capitated plans and high-deductible plans). Congress recognized that it would be a hard sell to persuade many of the elderly to choose managed care. Furthermore, it would be very costly to provide sufficient incentives for private plans to accept the oldest and sickest Medicare beneficiaries. Instead, Congress proposed a much meeker alternative. Beneficiaries would simply be given more options in addition to traditional fee-for-service Medicare. These additional options, called MedicarePlus plans, would be paid a premium by Medicare.

Rather than letting beneficiaries loose to find what they could in a private market, Medicare would require participating plans to cover all Medicare services. Plans that offered additional services could charge subscribers additional premiums. Offering additional plans, would not, by itself, reduce Medicare spending. Few beneficiaries were likely to choose alternative plans and Medicare would not save much money even if they did. If plans were able to offer services for less than the premium amounts, all savings would be returned to beneficiaries in the form of more generous benefits.

In order to guarantee savings that the Congressional Budget Office would count against the budget deficit, the congressional plan had to limit per capita payments for MedicarePlus premiums. Medicare payments for these plans would be allowed to grow only at prespecified rates roughly equal to those selected as cap rates under the Clinton plan. At the same time, Congress proposed significant cuts in payments to doctors, hospitals, laboratories, and other providers under the traditional Medicare fee-for-service program. These cuts, which take the form of fee reductions, make up the bulk of the savings from the plan (Congressional Budget Office 1995). Again, both the magnitude and the form of these cuts resembles those in the Clinton plan.

It is the last element of the congressional plan that most clearly illustrates the effect of the budget deficit on the making of health policy. Like the Clinton administration, the Republican Congress could not accept the chance that their reform would not yield the savings they had promised. On top of the savings achieved by reducing payments, they added a fail-safe mechanism that would automatically reduce Medicare spending. This mechanism would adjust payment rates in the fee-for-service sector to ensure that budget targets were met (Congressional Budget Office 1995). In both appearance and effect, the fail-safe mechanism operated like the global budgets in the Clinton plan.

8 ///

Financing Health Care: A Proposal

The failure of the Clinton health plan leaves the United States without a formal system of universal medical care coverage and with an increasingly threatened informal safety net. Federal, state, and local governments, facing mounting budget pressures, are hoping that a greater reliance on managed care will allow them to maintain quality while they cut back on spending in public health insurance programs. Private cost containment efforts have sharpened competition among hospitals, weakening their financial ability to provide care to those without insurance. These public and private efforts can save money in government budgets and workers' wallets today. They cannot stop health care costs from rising in the future.

Health care costs will rise because medicine will be able to do more for people. Most Americans will grumble about the increase in costs but they will pay for more care, just as they have for the past 65 years. People who cannot see well will gladly work more hours to fund better eyesight, when medical advances enable them to do so. People who cannot walk will willingly move to smaller dwellings if doctors offer them a chance to purchase physical mobility in exchange. More people will undergo screening tests—and costly treatment—for cancer when those tests become less uncomfortable. People at risk of strokes will skip vacations to buy artery cleaning that promises to diminish these risks. People in pain will sacrifice much of their other consumption for respite. People whose incomes rise will buy more health care without giving up anything they have today.

Simply put, health care costs will continue to rise. Governments, however, will find it ever more difficult to pay the cost of care for people in public programs. Once again, the Congress will thrill to the cries of fraud, waste, and abuse. Policy analysts will testify that one or another strategy will save billions of dollars while providing better care. If past history is a guide, the outcome will be more regulation combined with a further deterioration in the regular stream of funding of care for the poor. Yet, surprisingly, this outcome is avoidable. The problem of funding care for the poor when costs increase is one that people once knew how to solve.

Before continuing, I want to make it clear that funding care for the poor is not the only problem facing the health care system. As I have pointed out, the current system as well as medicalist and marketist reform proposals all suffer from a variety of further problems. But funding care for the poor is a particularly pervasive and intractable problem. Nevertheless, as I describe below, a straightforward solution can be incorporated into either type of health reform approach.

How America Once Cross-Subsidized Health Care

In better days long ago, before health insurance and government regulations, hospitals and physicians served their communities, or so the popular imagination holds. Neighborhood doctors treated everyone, varying their fees according to patients' abilities to pay for treatment. They served the most impoverished patients as an act of charity, charging nothing or only token fees. The local doctor might have been more deferential and zealous in responding to the needs of wealthier patients, and he (seldom she, back then) would probably recommend more costly treatments for them; but the poor got treatment too. Communities constructed hospitals to provide care for all, charging more to patients who could pay more and financing the care of the poor from the excess revenues earned from treating wealthier patients (Stevens 1989). Again, the poor might have worse accommodations, in public wards rather than private rooms, but everyone who needed treatment would get it.

Wealthier patients did not object to overpaying for their care—either because they approved of the charitable objectives that necessitated that overpayment or, more likely, because most wealthy patients had no other place to go. With only a very few doctors and hospitals in a community, paying patients would have been hard pressed to find medical services at lower prices even if they lacked charitable impulses. Physicians and hospitals could use their monopoly power to extract more dollars from paying patients.[1] Some used those extra dollars to fund care for the poor (although many others undoubtedly did not).[2]

The kind of cost shifting that once happened in mythical America provided a remarkably good solution to the problem of redistributing medical care. Charging more to paying patients to subsidize care for the poor meant that health care funding kept pace with improvements in health care technology. The poor always received less care than did paying patients, but relative levels of spending did not change over time. Paying patients implicitly took the poor into account when they made their own health care decisions. Choosing more care meant paying more directly and paying more in subsidies. Only care that was valued as much as the sum of direct costs and overcharges was purchased. That is, without necessarily recognizing it, paying patients would only buy care for themselves if they were also willing to buy more care for the poor.

Technological Change: Cost Shifting, Medicalist Models, and Marketist Models

In such a cost-shift world, the level of medical spending and the rate and nature of medical-technology diffusion are endogenously determined and take equity concerns into account. Individual consumers, through their own spending decisions, determine whether more money should be spent on medical care for themselves and for others. This endogeneity contrasts both with the central determination of spending levels required by the medicalist model and the disjunction between individual choices and equity concerns implicit in the marketist model.

In a medicalist system, a tax on income subsidizes health spending. If health care costs rise as a share of national income, the government must raise marginal tax rates to fund the new spending. Governments must weigh the political and economic costs of such increases against the benefits of higher health spending. Over time the level and pace in change of spending that a sensible government would choose would fall below the private spending choices of higher-income people.[3] Equity can most easily be attained at relatively low levels of spending (see Lindsay 1969).

If government sets the overall level of spending, the gap between that level and privately desired spending will increase as innovations occur. The system will appear "underfunded" and those who can afford it will seek ways around prohibitions on private care. A two-tiered system will emerge, complete with disparities between private and public care that offend the medicalists' egalitarian views about health care.

Marketists give most of the decision-making power in the system to individuals, as in the cost-shift world. When innovations occur, each person decides whether to buy them or not, and each person finances them by working harder or giving up other goods and services. Here too, however, decisions about spending on the poor must be made through the political system. Although a much smaller share of health care spending would be tax financed, this model, too, would have to balance political and economic concerns about raising taxes and diverting money to fund health spending. As the tax costs of funding health care rise, the economic consequences of allowing costs in the public sector to rise will also increase. A rational government would not permit costs of care to rise as quickly in the public sector as in the private sector. With public costs growing more slowly, the relative level of care provided to those in publicly funded programs would decline (Newhouse 1994).

Technological progress over time will bring a growing disparity between privately purchased care and publicly funded care. The initial desire for a more equitable system will be squashed by the burden of the continually rising taxes needed to finance it. If the interest in equity resurfaces, the political response will be to control the system by intervening in the private market. This is exactly the pattern proposed in the Clinton plan: markets would be permitted to work only if public funding could keep up with them.

A Theory of Health Care Redistribution

Redistributive concerns in the United States focus on ensuring a more egalitarian distribution of health services than would occur without intervention in the market. Rather than treating health care as one component in a bundle of money, goods, and services provided to the poor, Americans have a specific interest in the distribution of medical services. The goal of providing and maintaining a more equitable distribution of medical services can be achieved either by pulling down the level of care of the prosperous or by raising the level of care for the indigent. Either approach will narrow the gap.

One side of the gap has been addressed on a theoretical level in previous economic analyses. Analysts of the economics of redistribution in health care have argued that society's interest in providing medical services to the poor can generate what economists call an externality— an effect on people who neither receive nor provide the services (Lindsay 1969; Pauly 1971). If people care about providing the indigent with health services, then public financing of those services has two kinds of benefits. First, it benefits the poor directly because they get health care. Second, it generates external benefits (externalities) to non-indigent people who are made better off by knowing that the poor have received care. Even people who play no part in these transactions, neither paying taxes nor receiving free health services, may benefit psychically from the provision of these services. The existence of these externalities provides an economic justification for public financing of some level of health care for the indigent.

By the same token, those who value an equitable distribution of health resources are affected by private decisions by the nonpoor to increase their own health spending. More health spending by the prosperous widens the gap between rich and poor in just the same way that an increase in spending on the poor narrows it (Lindsay 1969). The private decision to pursue more costly and aggressive treatment affects the well-being of *all* Americans by changing the notion of what constitutes adequate care for the indigent.

In practical terms, an improvement in the quality of care selected by the prosperous has significant social implications in an environment that values health service equity. A private decision to increase spending must have one of two undesirable consequences: either health care equity will decline or the government must increase spending on the public program. In the latter case, balancing the government's budget will mean either reducing spending on other valuable public programs or raising tax rates and triggering the economic distortions associated with higher rates. Generating an equitable distribution is simply much more costly at higher levels of health spending than at lower levels.[4] Thus private decisions about spending levels, which appear to be of no economic interest to third parties, can have substantial public implications.

The cost-shifting model internalized this externality. Higher-income patients paid more for services than did lower-income patients. The system explicitly redistributed health services. In effect, the financing system generated cross-subsidies between those who could afford to purchase care and those who could not.

Recent innovations in the treatment of myocardial infarction (heart attacks) using drugs called thrombolytic agents provide a vivid example of the problems involved in addressing these externalities in today's health care sector as well as under a medicalist or a marketist reform. In late 1987 the U.S. Food and Drug Administration approved a new thrombolytic drug, t-PA, for the treatment of heart attacks. Early studies suggested that t-PA was somewhat more effective in reducing mortality from heart attacks than was another recently introduced thrombolytic drug, streptokinase. Streptokinase, though, costs only one-tenth as much as t-PA (Burke 1993).

In 1988 the government of Ontario, under a medicalist model, decided not to reimburse hospitals for the costs of using t-PA for any patients with heart attacks. The government argued that data on the effectiveness of the drug were quite incomplete and that the benefits did not yet appear to justify the added costs. Canadian health system rules prohibited hospitals from accepting payments from patients who wanted to receive the drugs. Faced with limited funding, hospitals restricted the use of t-PA and a survey found that doctors administered streptokinase about three times more frequently than t-PA (Naylor et al. 1990). In the United States, under a (more or less) marketist model, use of t-PA grew rapidly after its initial approval. Surveys in 1989 found that 60 to 80 percent of physicians primarily used t-PA rather than streptokinase in their practices (Brody et al. 1991; Lessler and Avins 1992). Economic considerations did affect the choice of drugs. Doctors in health maintenance organizations were much more likely to use streptokinase than were other doctors (Lessler and Avins 1992). Uninsured patients, Medicaid patients, and patients in public hospitals were also relatively more likely to receive streptokinase than they were t-PA, but, according to survey responses, even these patients were likely to receive t-PA about half the time.[5]

In Canada the introduction of t-PA meant an increase in the gap between the amount of health care people would choose for themselves and the amount provided under the public program. While many Canadians would have voluntarily selected lower-cost care and chosen streptokinase over t-PA, many others undoubtedly would have spent more to receive the slightly better drug. Under the medicalist system, this choice was entirely barred. Canada avoided the inequality associated with higher levels of use by higher-income people, but at the cost of making this group worse off without making anyone else better off.[6]

In the United States, the rapid spread of t-PA brought both a further divergence in the quality of care received by uninsured, Medicaid, and privately insured patients and an increase in the costs of programs that provide care to the poor (since some uninsured and Medicaid patients did receive t-PA). Privately insured patients who chose the drug, though, had no incentive to consider these further consequences. Private choices led to effects on third parties that were not taken into account by those who made the choices. Those who strongly valued health equity were made worse off by the increased divergence in the nature of care; those who pay taxes were made worse off by the increased cost of care. These negative effects can be seen most clearly in the case of heart attack patients who had joined HMOs. These patients bore a double burden: they were less likely to receive t-PA themselves than were those who chose more costly insurance plans, but they still paid the higher taxes associated with financing t-PA for indigent patients.

Neither the United States nor the Canadian system gets it right. The Canadian restriction on the use of a costly drug made those who would have chosen the drug worse off, without in any direct way benefiting those who could not afford the drug. The American system allows private decisions to have haphazard, unconsidered effects on the publicly funded health system—effects that drive up costs and reduce equity. Neither system does what the American goal of health redistribution suggests it should do: redistribute health care from those who choose a lot to those who cannot afford enough.

A Model for Financing Health Care

In today's health care marketplace, the mythical golden era of cost shifting, if it ever did exist, cannot be resurrected. Doctors and hospitals compete energetically for business and cannot compel well-to-do patients to pay extra for services. Managed-care organizations solicit bids from hospitals and use price as an element in their contracting. Hospitals and physicians who hope to find business cannot charge more than competitors do. In most parts of the country, the power of physicians and hospitals to charge extrahigh prices to certain patients to offset discounts for others has disappeared.

The structure of the health services industry has also changed in ways that make informal cross-subsidies impossible to resurrect. The proliferation and diffusion of services that exist in today's market, including freestanding diagnostic and surgical clinics and legions of local specialists and subspecialists, mean that many physicians and health service facilities do not serve a diverse cross-section of the population. Patients spend only a day or two in the hospital, not long enough to feel a special connection to the particular facility. Many physicians treat only rich people or only poor people, thus eliminating the possibility of charging more to some to provide care for others. The very existence of publicly provided insurance financed by taxes may reduce charitable donations to hospitals (Sloan et al. 1990).

Although the possibility of returning to America's mythical age of health care financing has disappeared, the appeal of the myth endures. People who benefit from the miracles of medicine should, it suggests, share their good fortune.[7] Hospitals exploit this idea when they solicit former patients to endow new equipment, clinics, or buildings. They anticipate that gratitude for treatment received will fortify the prospective donors' charitable impulses and generate donations from them. Anecdotal evidence suggests that this strategy is quite successful.[8]

Can the benefits of a cost-shifting system be resurrected? I believe that they can, through a two-pronged approach: taxing health care spending and redistributing funds according to income.

Raising Funds

A tax on health care providers would address three concerns. First, it would provide funding to finance health care for the poor. Second, it would force the more affluent to take into account the way their health purchase decisions affect the level of health care that society chooses to provide to the poor. Finally, in so doing, it would make the level of sustainable national health spending an outcome of a private decision-making process, not a constraint imposed arbitrarily from above. Health care financing would mimic the dynamic nature of health care itself. Health care revenues would rise when costs rise.

The health tax would be levied on all suppliers of health services: doctors, hospitals, freestanding surgical centers, pharmacists, insurers, and managed-care companies. Services paid by insurance would be taxed through a levy on premiums, and services financed through out-of-pocket payments would be taxed directly. Eventually, most of the cost of this tax would be passed along to service purchasers in the form of higher prices.[9] All services would be taxed at a single, unchanging tax rate. If people, on average, chose to purchase more costly services, the tax would yield more revenue, but the rate would not change.

People who chose more costly health care would pay more in taxes (a flat percentage of a higher price) than would those who were more frugal in their health care choices. In the example of the choice of t-PA and streptokinase described above, the prices of both drugs would reflect the same tax rate, but the price of t-PA would include a higher absolute dollar amount of tax revenue than would the price of streptokinase. Purchasers of t-PA would contribute more to the provision of thrombolytic drugs (or other care) to the indigent than would users of streptokinase. Total consumption of thrombolytic drugs (measured in terms of dollar-valued units) would decline as a consequence of the tax.

Tax revenues would be used to subsidize health services for people with low incomes. The effect of the subsidies would be to provide more health services to those who could not otherwise afford them, benefiting both the recipients of services and those concerned about the equitable distribution of medical care. The amount of the subsidy provided would depend on the amount of tax revenue collected. As health care costs rose, more revenue would be collected and the per capita subsidy would rise. If high-income purchasers became more frugal in their health care choices or if technological improvements led to reductions in the cost of care (see Schwartz 1994), subsidies would decline. The revenues raised to redistribute health care would wane and wax along with health spending.

From a tax policy perspective, a tax within the health services sector would have few distortionary effects. If my reasoning above is correct, health care usage generates externalities in the form of growing in-

equities; a tax on health care would, in effect, force health care purchasers to consider the impact of their decisions on others.[10] They are
likely to respond by spending less on health care out-of-pocket and less
on health insurance (Phelps 1976). One likely way for consumers to
reduce spending on health care and health insurance is to choose plans
that incorporate more restrictions on service use, such as HMOs or
high-deductible traditional insurance plans.

How large is the health care consumption externality? Today, the
typical uninsured individual receives about 60 percent as much care as
does the average insured person (adjusting for health status).[11] The
fact that that figure has remained roughly constant since about 1957
suggests that it may represent underlying social preferences about the
relationship between minimum adequate care and average privately financed care. A one-dollar increase in health consumption by an upper-
income American appears to lead people to increase the minimally adequate bundle of care available to the poor by 60 cents. This concern
about assuring minimally adequate health consumption may encompass
the population with incomes below 200 percent of the poverty line,
about one-third of the U.S. population. Under these assumptions, a
health tax rate of 30 percent would correct for the external effects of
health care consumption. If the extent of redistribution desired was
lower or the population of concern was smaller, the tax rate would be
correspondingly smaller too.[12]

The health tax rate should be constant across the nation. In areas
where health costs are high, the tax would collect more revenue. Unlike
financing proposals that focus exclusively on the decisions of individuals
at the margin, the flat health tax proposal encourages regions to make
considered decisions about the average cost of care. Areas that chose
to raise the cost and quality of care by building elaborate new health
facilities could do so, but they would pay more in taxes. Just as the
health tax would force individuals to consider the broader implications
of their health care choices, the tax would encourage states and localities to consider the full costs of their health planning decisions. A single
national rate would avoid the problem of a "race to the bottom"
among states and localities. By maintaining a single tax rate across the
nation, jurisdictions would compete only by reducing the cost of care
for all, not by cutting services to their poorest residents.

In its effects, the health tax I propose is the mirror image of the existing tax treatment of employer-provided health insurance. The tax treatment of health insurance gives people an incentive to consume more health care; the health tax would give them incentives to consume less care. The current tax treatment provides the most government support to high-income taxpayers who choose costly care; the health tax imposes the smallest burden on those who choose frugal plans. The tax treatment of health insurance shifts the burden of health care spending from regions with costly utilization patterns to regions with thrifty ones; the health tax ties costs to the region in which they are incurred. The tax treatment of health insurance drains government coffers when health costs rise, making it ever more difficult to finance care for the indigent; the health tax replenishes the treasury when costs rise, making it easier to finance care for the indigent.

Unfortunately, simply abolishing the tax treatment of employer-provided health insurance benefits would not achieve the goals of the health tax. Eliminating this special tax treatment would reduce the effects on government budgets of increases in private health costs, but it would not generate a stream of new revenues to offset the costs of those who require subsidies. Eliminating the tax treatment is an important step toward developing a sustainable financing system, but it does not take us far enough.

The need to generate a politically acceptable stream of new revenues has led many state lawmakers to consider using provider taxes to fund health care benefits. A number of states have proposed financing some care through taxes on hospitals or providers (for example, see Crittenden 1993 for a description of the Washington State plan and Leichter 1993 for a description of the Minnesota plan). Premium and provider taxes are used in many states to raise funds for high-risk insurance pools and other redistributive functions. In New York State, uncompensated care and graduate medical education in hospitals is financed through a 13 percent surcharge on hospital care paid only by those with private commercial insurance (not Blue Cross coverage). The tax raises over $3 billion annually (Alpha Center 1995). The health tax proposal described above provides a rationale for this increasingly popular kind of state health care financing.

A health tax could raise a substantial amount of money for redistribution. A 30 percent tax on the $782.5 billion Americans spent on health care in 1993 might reduce health care spending by 5 percent and would raise $220 billion on the remainder. The tax would not raise as much as current health-related taxes. It would, however, cover all current Medicaid spending, all Medicare spending for seniors with incomes below twice the poverty line, and would leave $35 billion toward coverage for the uninsured.[13]

A health tax would not have a substantial effect on national health spending. Studies of the effect of eliminating the tax treatment of health insurance show that this increase in insurance costs would reduce health spending by less than 10 percent (Marquis and Buchanan 1994). A tax on health spending might have even smaller effects, because it would not lead people to substitute out-of-pocket payments for health insurance coverage. But as I indicated in Chapter 4, the evidence suggests that, as a nation, Americans can afford to buy more health care if they choose to do so. The advantage of the health tax is that it generates a level of health spending that the nation can support. The level of health care that is freely chosen under a health tax represents both the amount people wish to purchase for themselves and the amount the nation can spend on the care of those who cannot afford to pay to maintain a given level of health equity. The health tax transforms the debate about cost containment from an argument about the right amount of health care for the nation to a more focused discussion about the level of health services equity that is desirable.

Disbursing Funds

Like many other health reform proposals, the health tax would disburse funds according to income. While raising funds through a tax on health care will have minimal distortionary effects, disbursing funds according to income will have unavoidable distortionary implications. If you can receive equally good health care whether you work or not, the health subsidy will reduce incentives to work. The disincentive to work is greatest if the subsidy is phased out sharply. For example, if everyone with an income under $20,000 receives free health insurance and everyone with an income over $19,999 must pay the full cost, those earning $19,999 would sensibly reject offers of additional work that would cost them their free health insurance coverage. These distortionary effects are identical to those that plague other income-related redistributional programs.

In this program, as in others, distortionary effects can be minimized through careful design choices. First, the subsidy can be phased out gradually. A gradual phaseout, however, increases the number of people covered by the program and its cost. Second, eligibility for subsidies should be limited to income alone. Promising health insurance subsidies to people on the basis of age or other characteristics will increase the size of the tax, the size of the program, and the distortionary effects of the program. Finally, distortionary effects can be diminished by limiting the generosity of the free health insurance benefit. A limited benefit will reduce the number of people who receive health care subsidies. Increasing the level of equity in the system means increasing the number of people who receive health care subsidies.

What Would a Health Tax Do for Equity?

The health tax takes health care redistribution outside the debate about overall government priorities. The decision about how equitable to make health services delivery is independent of any decisions about social equity generally. This partition is consistent with the historic separation of programs that provide health care from those that address the income needs of the poor. As the history of medical transfer programs such as Medicare and Medicaid suggests, people do not use health transfers as a vehicle to make the poor better off overall. Rather, the transfers are employed to keep the distribution of health services relatively equitable.

Indeed, under today's financing system, society's interests in improving the lot of the poor and its interests in the equity of health services are actually in opposition. Achieving the one often means sacrificing the other. For example, the desire to maintain funding for the Medicaid program in the face of rising health costs has led to cutbacks in funding for other programs that serve the poor, particularly programs that provide cash assistance. Increasing Medicaid funding while reducing cash payments motivates most poor people to use more health services than they would choose if they received all transfers in a single cash payment. A few poor people (those with medical problems) may be made better off, and it may comfort higher-income people to know that the poor receive important medical services, but if the services come at the expense of cash assistance, they hurt, rather than benefit, the vast majority of the poor themselves. By recognizing that society's interest in health services redistribution is distinct from its interests in other kinds of redistribution, the health tax removes the question of funding health care for the poor from the broader issue of assistance to the poor. This will enable policymakers to devote appropriate attention to the general needs of the poor, undistracted by surges in health care costs.

In this sense, the health tax runs counter to the original marketist idea that health care redistribution is simply a politically feasible way of achieving a more equitable distribution of social resources in general. Treating health care as an element in overall resource redistribution has, until now, had the perverse effect of further impoverishing the poor when health care costs rise. Society has an interest in the redistribution of health care, but liberals cannot piggyback general redistribution on that interest. Health care redistribution can transfer health care resources to achieve a more equitable distribution of these resources, but it cannot successfully do more than that.

The health tax recognizes that health care redistribution cannot achieve general social equity. Indeed, its design also embeds a degree of inequality and means-testing into the distribution of health care itself. The health tax cannot and is not intended to generate a perfectly equal distribution of health services that reflects medically determined needs for services. But it can generate a perpetually rising level of adequate care for those in need, a level that improves as health care improves.

In Defense of a Multitiered Health Care System

The cost-shift world—and the health tax world—do not generate a perfectly equitable distribution of health care, as the medicalist model would. Rather, they generate a multitiered system of health care. Poor patients receive considerably less care, in less comfortable circumstances, than do those with more money. What do such inequities imply about health care?

The experience of a broad range of other countries with very different health systems suggests that it is possible to provide people with a fairly high level of basic health care for half as much as the amount spent (per capita) in the United States. In general, other countries do not achieve these results by making difficult and explicit rationing decisions such as denying services to people in certain categories (for example, those over seventy) or prohibiting the use of new treatments. Rather, they achieve their results by slowing the introduction and diffusion of new technologies, concentrating costly procedures at a limited number of centers, delaying access to expensive care, and using more generalists and fewer specialists.

It is important to recognize that the costs of these strategies are real ones. As recent studies comparing Canada and the United States suggest, patients in cost-contained systems may experience more discomforts and delays than patients who spend more money. Delays in access to high-technology care will, in some instances, lead to worse health for particular patients than might have been achieved through speedier treatment. Most evidence, however, suggests that on average these differences in access to costly services have minimal effects on overall physiological health.

Some would even argue that these expenditure-reducing strategies have benefits as well as drawbacks. Requiring patients to wait for treatment certainly imposes costs on the patients, but it allows higher use of existing health care capacity and may lead some patients to decide to forgo treatment after thinking through their situation more carefully. Concentrating procedures in a few centers adds to patient inconvenience, but it helps to ensure that those performing procedures have more experience. Reducing the pace at which new technology is introduced means some people are deprived of procedures that might help them, but others are spared procedures that turn out to do more harm than good. Using more generalists may mean that doctors have less knowledge of the latest developments in a field, but they may be better at managing the patient as a person.

While allowing those who could afford it to avoid discomforts and delays, a multitiered system would guarantee a level of care to all that was equivalent in cost to that provided in most other countries. The cost-saving strategies employed by other national health systems could readily be (and are being) adopted by frugal managed-care companies. These companies, operating on a fixed budget, could offer adequate but low-intensity care to those who cannot afford more. Those who really care about having their knee operation next week and not in two months, or seeing a subspecialist rather than a general practitioner, or being treated in a modern, high-technology local facility rather than a central hospital can pay more for these valued benefits.

Under a health tax, this group would also contribute more to care for the poor. A health tax would not produce a two-tiered health system: it would produce a multitiered health system. Some people would receive care at the defined adequacy standard, others would buy somewhat more care than that, and some would choose superluxury care. No one would go without care, but some people would receive more and probably better care than others. The world of widely diverging incomes would continue to generate an unequal distribution of health care. But the tax could be relied on to produce revenues sufficient to assure that the lowest level of spending was in constant relationship to higher levels of spending. A gap between the rich and poor would remain, but it would not widen. The quality of care available to the poor would rise as the quality of care purchased by the affluent rose.

The health tax can permit inequality because it avoids a common concern about nonuniversal programs. Policy proposals often call for an equal, universal benefit because proponents fear that without middle-class support the program they are pitching will eventually be underfunded. The health tax would generate a growing stream of income over time without requiring increases in tax rates. While the health tax will not bring equality, it will proscribe growing inequality.

How Would a Health Tax Work in Practice?

A health tax and subsidy program would generate a health care system that falls somewhere between a marketist and a medicalist model. Health care would not be distributed perfectly equitably, but equity considerations would enter all decisions. A health tax could be incorporated into either a marketist or medicalist system of health reform.

Consider, for example, a very simple marketist reform that gives currently uninsured low-income people health insurance vouchers and has them seek care in the marketplace. This kind of reform might also include the development of insurance-purchasing organizations and a system of risk adjustment to respond to adverse selection and risk selection problems (see, for an example, the Bush health care proposal, described in CEA 1992). In this model, the health tax would raise revenues for vouchers for redistribution. The existing Medicare program would continue, but Medicaid might be incorporated into the voucher system. In order to fund this new voucher program, the health tax would have had to raise about $150 billion in 1993.[14] A 30 percent tax on all private health insurance and out-of-pocket payments would raise this sum (while the income taxes and other levies now used to fund Medicaid and uncompensated care could be eliminated). Note that incorporating the health tax into this marketist proposal does draw it part of the way toward the medicalist camp. Funding health care through a tax on health ties the spending decisions of higher-income Americans to those of lower-income Americans in a way that a proposal based on other taxes would not. At the same time, the health tax protects the market from the excessive regulation and pressure for systemwide cost containment that otherwise accompany increases in the cost of government programs.

A health tax could also be used as an element of a more medicalist, single-payer health program like the Canadian health care system. Under a health tax proposal, hospitals, physicians, and other providers would be allowed to opt out of the existing fee schedule, forming a separate private system of care. The private system could be reimbursed by private health insurance or out-of-pocket payments.[15] All services rendered in this private system would be taxed at the health tax rate. The funds raised from the health tax would be used to enrich the existing public system.

Suppose, for example, that 25 percent of the population chose to participate in the private system and initially spent an average of $1,000 in that program. A 30 percent health tax rate would ensure that for the next 20 years average spending by those who opted out would be no more than 30 percent higher than per capita spending in the public system, even if spending in the private system grew twice as quickly as spending financed by income taxes in the public system.[16] Furthermore, a 30 percent tax rate on private spending would allow the total funding of the public system to grow a little faster (about 0.1 percent per capita faster) than it would otherwise. Unlike other two-tier models, equity in this system would grow if more people opted into the private sector or if those who used the private sector reduced their spending in the public sector. Rather than leading to further underfunding of the public sector, under a health tax these changes would reduce average disparities in spending and lead to faster growth of the public sector. Again, adding a taxed private sector to a medicalist system would draw it part of the way into the marketist camp by introducing some inequity into the system. At the same time, by reducing cost pressure, a health tax could be used to protect medicalist interests in the integrity of the public sector of the system.

Conclusion

The health tax model addresses only one of the many problems inherent in marketist or medicalist health reforms. But the problem of funding the system over time, the problem that the health tax is intended to address, in practice eclipses all the other failures of regulatory design. Without money, there can be no real health reform.

Any health system reform will be undone without a stable, growing source of funding. A medicalist reform, faced with diminishing resources, will further constrain the growth of services. Attempts to save money will lead to increased micromanagement of medical practice, undermining the medicalist interest in empowering physicians. Constraints will also squeeze the political consensus that maintains the system. Wealthier people will opt out and their support for tax financing will diminish.

A marketist-oriented reform, like the managed competition considered by the Clinton administration, will also be undone by funding woes. With health care spending rising more rapidly than incomes or economic output, a broad-based tax—which is a tax on overall economic activity—will over time fall short. The government can, for a time, broaden the tax base, as it did in funding the Medicare trust fund, or it can raise rates; but ultimately, increasing costs will require the government to take an active hand in forcing costs down. Any public program thus raises the specter of more and more government cost containment—with government regulation eventually intruding into the private health care sector.

Everybody wants health care reform, but nobody wants to pay for it. The rift between people's charitable sentiments toward the poor and their proprietary feelings toward their pocketbooks has been the bane of health reform. But this time the public is right. None of the solutions advanced to address the problem of health care redistribution up to now will work in the long run, and Americans should reject all of them.

One solution, emphasized in recent debates over the Clinton plan and Medicare reform, is to apply the efficiency gains from reforming the system to fund care. But although improving the system can save money, it simply will not save enough to cover the costs of care ten or even five years from now. Efficiency savings are onetime-only events. Given the dynamic nature of medical change, they cannot provide a stable base for funding care for the uninsured in the future.

A second way to fund health reform is by imposing constraints on existing public programs. If Medicare and Medicaid grow more slowly than currently projected, the additional revenues that would have been needed to fund these programs can be diverted to the uninsured. Unfortunately, there is little evidence to suggest that cost growth in Medicare and Medicaid have been substantially different from cost growth in the private sector. Over time, achieving lower rates of growth in these public programs would yield a widening gap between the quality of publicly funded and privately funded care. That gap could be eliminated only by making the private system grow more slowly too. Making the private system grow more slowly means restraining private spending decisions. That is neither politically feasible nor economically desirable.

Hardheaded reformers assert that the public should be made to bite the bullet. Those who want universal coverage should be prepared to pay for it through higher broad-based taxes. Here too, the public says no and the public is right. Broad-based taxes are not the answer to health reform. In the long run, they just won't work. With health costs growing faster than the economy as a whole, broad-based taxes will not raise the stream of revenue needed to assure that care for the poor keeps pace with improvements in care for everyone else. Either the gap between rich and poor will widen, or tax rates will have to be continually increased.

The health tax model I propose can provide a long-term basis for funding health care equity. It takes the growing level of private health consumption and redirects part of it to fund health care for the poor. It is a revenue source that will grow along with the need for the revenues. Finally, a provider tax fits popular perceptions about how health care should work by making the beneficiaries of modern medical care share its rewards. It updates the mythical vision of community health care to correspond with the realities of medical care today. It maintains a level of equality in the distribution of health services. It generates a level of health care spending that both the nation and the government can afford—today and twenty years from now.

Notes

1. Introduction

1. Immediately after Clinton's speech, two-thirds of those polled approved of the plan (Brownstein 1993). Senate minority leader Dole recommended that Republicans work with President Clinton to produce a health care bill (Nelson 1993).

2. Insurance companies price policies to individuals based on individual health risks and to small groups based on average risk in the group. Most large group policies do not have an insurance-risk component. Insurance companies simply administer the health care package. In such cases the "price" of insurance is the average cost incurred by the members of the group.

3. Insurance coverage may have been falling well before 1988. Changes in the way that data sources count the uninsured (especially a change in the definition in 1987) make it difficult to say with certainty.

4. Unfortunately, the amounts Americans say they would be willing to pay for universal coverage do not come close to the sums needed. In 1993, 41 percent said they would be willing to pay $480 more in taxes per year for national health insurance that would cover everyone and eliminate all other payments (Jacobs and Shapiro 1993). By my calculations the actual per capita cost of health care for this benefit is about five times that high.

5. The group was led by Paul Starr and Walter Zelman. Their article "A Bridge to Compromise: Competition under a Budget" (Starr and Zelman 1993) provides a description of the plan they devised.

6. Starr 1982 and Rothman 1993 discuss the role of health care lobbies in defeating earlier reform efforts.

7. For a discussion of these criticisms, see Fallows 1995.

8. Those who did read the plan uncovered enforcement and regulatory mechanisms that rarely figured in public discussions, and this prompted a sense that the plan was riddled with hidden dangers and booby traps. See Elizabeth McCaughey's very effective if, in many respects, inaccurate critique in *The New Republic* (McCaughey 1994).

9. Small, low-wage-businesses would pay a much smaller share of payroll for health insurance than would larger businesses. Small, low-wage-business payments would be capped, while the largest employers would receive no subsidies at all. This subsidy structure was roundly criticized by economists for generating substantial distortions of the labor market. Over time this system could have been expected to lead to a concentration of low-wage workers in the smallest firms.

10. The rising private share of health care spending in Great Britain and the increasing interest in privatizing part of the system in Canada suggest that reform of financing mechanisms will be needed even in centrally constrained health care systems.

2. Medicalists and Marketists

1. Political conservatives, whose ideological disposition favors smaller government, are often also marketists.

2. These innovations would probably also lead the rate of technological change itself to conform more closely to the theoretically optimal level (Baumgardner 1991).

3. All figures are in 1991 dollars.

3. The Illusion of Inefficiency

1. These calculations are based on the Department of Commerce 1981 and 1993 *Current Population Survey* data tapes. In 1980, 22 percent of those employed in health care were in administrative-support positions. In 1992, 26 percent were in such positions. The fraction who were health professionals did not change over the decade.

2. I exclude lawyers employed in law offices and accountants employed in accounting offices from these calculations. Looking at legal and accounting services only (excluding investment banking), administrative-support personnel increased by 446,000, or 74 percent, between 1980 and 1992.

3. Staffing increased between 1980 and the date indicated in parentheses in Austria (1990), Canada (1985), Denmark (1990), Finland (1990), Germany (1989), Greece (1990), Italy (1989), Japan (1990), the Netherlands (1990), Norway (1989), New Zealand (1985), Portugal (1990), Spain (1989), and the United Kingdom (1985). Staffing declined in France between 1980 and 1990 but increased between 1975 and 1990 and between 1985 and 1990.

4. The real difference in national health spending (expressed in 1991 dollars) was $103.9 billion (CBO 1993c).

5. About $4 billion covers the compensation costs of 1 in 15 (1 in 25) of those actually injured. I assume that the cost of compensation is one-fourth as high for those not compensated. Then, the cost of compensating all those injured is ¼ × $4 billion × 14 [24] + $4 billion, or $18 [$28] billion.

6. Even this low figure is an enormous improvement over earlier practices. In 1976 only 12 physicians in the entire nation lost their licenses because of malpractice (Gaumer 1984).

7. The cost of capital invested by the government in a single-payer system also comes at a cost—the cost of withdrawing these funds from other valued investments. A proper cost comparison of single-payer and multipayer insurance systems should account for these forgone "profits." See, for example, Danzon 1992.

8. There may also be limited demand for insurance in these markets. The Robert Wood Johnson Foundation sponsored the development of lower-priced insurance packages that were made available to small businesses, but few businesses chose to buy the packages (McLaughlin and Zellers 1992). It is possible that innovation in the nature of the insurance product would have been more successful.

9. The presumed inferior quality of a system of for-profit insurers and managed-care companies when compared with one in which independent physicians are paid a fee for each service they render by a not-for-profit or public payer rests on the rather shaky presumption that physicians are inherently more ethical than other professionals and business people. If physicians are not unusually ethical, then for-profit insurers will not have a substantial effect on quality. Competition among insurers will reduce quality no more than competition does among providers. Either consumers can evaluate the quality of medicine—in which case they can evaluate the quality of managed-care plans—or they cannot. If not, they cannot assess the quality of independently practicing physicians either.

10. In the nursing-home market, for-profit operators also appear to be less costly (Frech 1985).

11. The ratio of physician incomes to average incomes ranges between 2.4 and 4.3 in Canada, Germany, and the United Kingdom.

12. Health services researchers have engaged in a long, inconclusive debate about the magnitude of such demand inducement. For a summary, see Folland, Goodman, and Stano 1993.

13. Ironically, federal health care reform may save the physician cartel. As provision of medical services becomes more organized, politicians, policy-

makers, and administrators will need a physician group to consult. The incentives to join and work through the cartel, rather than compete alone, will rise.

14. This pattern of rising returns during the 1980s to those with post-secondary education occurred in many developed countries and has been the subject of many studies. See, for example, Blackburn and Bloom 1995, and Katz, Loveman, and Blanchflower 1993.

15. Post-medical-school training ranges from three years for less specialized doctors to eight years for the most highly specialized groups (American Board of Medical Specialists 1991).

16. In 1988 surgeons earned 130 percent more than general practitioners, while other medical specialists earned 53 percent more than general practitioners (Pope and Schneider 1992).

17. The ratio of specialists to generalists has risen in several other OECD countries besides the United States (although the United States has far more specialists than any other OECD country).

18. The demand for specialty care is relatively price-inelastic, so a decline in price alone would lead to a decrease in total spending on specialty care.

19. Nevertheless, while policies for explicitly setting the mix of doctors in general care versus specialty care would be unlikely to achieve significant cost savings and could exacerbate existing discrepancies between the supply of and demand for specialists, it would be equally incorrect to believe that the current balance fully reflects underlying market forces. Graduate medical education in hospitals is subsidized by the federal government through the Medicare programs. The subsidy means that training in hospital-related specialties can be provided at lower cost than training in nonhospital specialties. In 1993 Medicare paid $1.3 billion to subsidize graduate medical education (CBO 1994b). By making it relatively less costly to become a specialist, such subsidies probably induce some physicians to continue their education and bias the physician workforce toward specialty care.

20. Computed by multiplying the number of physicians by their average earnings (according to AMA 1994 data).

21. If physicians responded by trying to make up that income, the decline in total spending would be even smaller.

22. This computation assumes that 30 percent of pacemaker implantations were equivocal.

23. Assessments of the relationship between variations in care and appropriateness of care can be easily biased by coding and other statistical problems (Phelps 1993). The Canadian/American comparison, however, which used two sets of criteria and two sets of rankers, should be less susceptible to this potential bias than single-criterion studies.

24. In 1991, 55 percent of medium and large private establishments capped

individual out-of-pocket expenses at or below $1,000 (Department of Labor 1991a).

25. Spending under the 25-percent-coinsurance policy is about 12 percent higher than spending under the 95-percent-coinsurance policy (Manning et al. 1987). Estimates in Feldman and Dowd suggest that a 95-percent-coinsurance policy is preferred to a 25-percent-coinsurance policy even if the marginal dollar of health spending is highly valued and prices are unaffected by the insurance change. The welfare gain, excluding risk reduction effects, of moving from a 25-percent-coinsurance policy to a 95-percent-coinsurance policy was approximately $340 per family in 1984 (based on estimates in Manning et al. 1987 and Feldman and Dowd 1991). This gain exceeds the loss from risk bearing estimated by Feldman and Dowd for moving from a policy with free care to a 95-percent-coinsurance policy, which, in turn, is an overestimate of the loss in risk bearing from moving from a policy with 25 percent coinsurance to one with 95 percent coinsurance.

26. A recent review of estimates by the CBO (1994d) suggests that the price elasticity of the demand for health insurance participation (buying or not buying insurance) generally equals or exceeds the price elasticity of demand for plan generosity. A 1 percent increase in the price of health insurance coverage would reduce participation by about 1 percent and reduce the generosity of plans among those remaining insured by 0.6 to 1 percent. Much of this reduction in generosity would come through elimination of vision care, dental care, and other low-risk benefits. These benefits, however, probably do not contribute much to the rate of increase in health care costs.

27. Such consumer preferences for low deductibles are not specific to New York State. In a 1986 sample of auto insurance purchasers in North Carolina, 42 percent bought coverage with a $100 deductible (Puelz and Snow 1994).

28. While the prices of these policies are not readily available, the New York State insurance department recommends raising deductible levels as a way of substantially reducing auto insurance premiums. The potential for moral hazard in the comprehensive-coverage market (which protects cars from vandalism, burglary, and fire damage) would seem to be substantial.

29. The 20 percent figure is my calculation based on the data in Berk and Monheit 1992; I do not recall the exact percentage quoted at the meeting.

30. U.S. per capita health spending in 1985 was $2,010; in Canada per capita spending was $1,546. U.S. per capita health spending in 1990 was $2,566, 27.8 percent higher. At this growth rate, if health spending in 1985 were reduced to the Canadian level, it would reach $1,976 per capita by 1990. Even if health spending grew at the somewhat slower Canadian rate, it would approach the 1985 level by 1993. (All figures are in 1991 dollars.)

4. Can We Afford More Health Care?

1. Note, however, that since the absolute level of costs was lower in other countries to begin with, this similarly rapid rate of growth means that the absolute gap in spending is widening.

2. In many of these countries, people hold private insurance policies that cover some share of these nonpublicly funded costs.

3. Between 1984 and 1991, costs rose from 4.9 percent of after-tax income to 5.1 percent of after-tax income. The entire change, however, occurred among the elderly, who spent 11.3 percent of their after-tax income on health care in 1984 and 12.2 percent in 1991. Among those under age sixty-five, the share of health spending remained constant at 4 percent (Cowan and McDonnell 1993).

4. Medicare and Medicaid spending in 1994 amounted to $246 billion, 3.7 percent of GDP. The CBO projects that in 2004, these costs will rise to $685 billion, 6.3 percent of GDP. If Medicare and Medicaid remained at 3.7 percent of GDP through 2004, the federal government's health spending in 2004 would be $285 billion lower, 80 percent of the projected 2004 deficit of $365 billion.

5. Data for earlier years used a somewhat different methodology and may not be comparable. The earlier figures suggest that spending on dogs and cats more than doubled (in real terms) between 1982 and 1987 (Wise 1984a, 1984b; Wise and Yang 1992, 1994). Projections from the American Veterinary Medicine Association suggest that health care spending on pets will grow by 84 percent between 1991 and 1998, again faster than the corresponding figures for human care (Wise and Yang 1994). The rapidly rising cost of veterinary care has in fact sparked a new interest in veterinary insurance.

6. The real growth rates of spending on nonprescription drugs and of GDP are as follows (based on data in Letsch et al. 1992, deflated using CPI):

Period	Annual growth rate of real GDP	Annual growth rate of real spending on nonprescription drugs
1960–1985	3.2%	4.1%
1980–1991	2.2%	3.9%

7. Examples of this pattern of rising (or flat) overall costs and declining unit costs include heart transplants, laparoscopic cholecystectomy, implantable defibrillators, and knee replacement (Woods et al. 1992; Legoretta et al. 1993; Smith 1993; Healy and Finn 1994).

8. If surgery costs were constant, the increase in bypass surgery in the pop-

ulation of men over sixty-five alone would have added almost $2 billion to health care costs.

9. Technology leads to similar rates of cost growth in other countries, but other countries save money by providing high-technology services to a smaller proportion of the population than does the United States. When a new technology is introduced, residents of other countries get access to it too, but since rates of use are lower than in the United States the absolute difference in cost grows.

10. The U.S. Census Bureau reports life expectancy both for men and for women and groups persons aged 80 to 84 in a separate category from those 85 and over. The United States ranks second to Greece among men 80 to 84; second to Cuba among men 85 and over; second to Canada among women 80 to 84, and highest among women 85 and over. One concern about these data is that the U.S. figures may reflect "survival of the fittest." Those Americans hardy enough to survive to 80 may be unusually strong.

11. Based on data from PROPAC 1993 and CEA 1994. Community-hospital admission rates in the United States in 1982 were 130 persons per 1,000 for those under 65 years old and 413 per 1,000 for those 65 or older. In 1992 the corresponding rates were 92 per 1,000 and 367 per 1,000. Average lengths of stay in 1982 were 7.6 days for those under 65 and 10.1 days for others. In 1992 the corresponding rates were 6.4 days and 8.3 days. The 1992 population consisted of 223 million people under 65 and 32 million people 65 or older.

12. As I noted in Chapter 3, the fact that insurance only covers monetary costs can lead to a bias in the pattern of technological change.

13. Luft's strongest estimates are for coronary artery bypass graft surgery. He finds that a 10 percent improvement in the quality of a hospital's outcomes with respect to this surgery would increase the probability of a patient selecting that hospital by 9.12 percent. A 10 percent reduction in distance to the hospital, though, would increase use by 13.72 percent. For the other procedures he considers, the distance effects outweigh the quality effects by much more.

14. One researcher estimated the carrying costs associated with queues for CABG surgery in British Columbia and found that they may amount to 0.6 percent of provincial GDP (Danzon 1992).

15. There was no apparent relationship between severity of patient's condition and length of wait in Canada. The existence of such a relationship would reduce carrying costs.

16. Some analysts note that courts often nullify insurance contract requirements that bar coverage for costly new technologies (Aaron 1993). Insurers, though, could save substantial sums without explicitly limiting access, simply by requiring patients to wait longer for services, as most government-run systems do.

17. American consumers spend a much smaller proportion of their incomes

on food than do Europeans. Here, too, differences in food spending outweigh differences in health care spending. In 1991, 14.9 percent of American consumption went to food (including alcohol), of which 9.4 percentage points were spent on food and alcohol at home. In France, food (excluding alcohol) accounted for 18.6 percent of consumption. In Germany, food and alcohol accounted for 19.5 percent of consumption. In Italy, food (excluding alcohol) accounted for 20.7 percent of consumption, and in the United Kingdom, food and alcohol at home accounted for 13.7 percent of consumption (Leyland 1990).

18. Reinhart counterargues that rising health spending can affect competitiveness because it draws down government spending on productive investments like education.

19. Between 1980 and 1990, average real per capita health spending increased 4.4 percent per year (CBO 1993c). Average real vendor payments per beneficiary in Medicaid increased 4.1 percent per year (DHHS 1993).

20. Part B expenditures in 1993 amounted to $56 billion, of which beneficiaries paid $14.5 billion. The federal deficit was $254.7 billion in 1993.

21. The countries with health insurance programs funded by general revenue are Canada, Italy, New Zealand, Spain, Sweden, and the United Kingdom (Hoffmeyer and McCarthy 1994).

22. For example, in 1980, after a 39 percent increase (in one year) in the price of gasoline, 45 percent of those polled supported a return to gas rationing (Gallup Poll, February 11, 1980).

23. At 0.8 percent, the growth in real per capita GDP excluding health care will be only half as high as the corresponding figure for the period 1960 to 1990 (Burner, Waldo, and McKusick 1992).

5. How Much to Whom?

1. In 1950, 9 to 12 percent of personal health expenditures were financed through loans (Serbein 1953).

2. My calculations, based on data in Berk and Monheit 1992, CBO 1993c, and CEA 1992; all figures are in 1991 dollars. Data on national health spending per capita were adjusted to reflect personal health spending, about 89 percent of national health expenditures (Letsch et al. 1992). After this adjustment, per capita health expenditures in 1963 were $626 (1991 dollars). In 1987 per capita personal health expenditures were $2,090 (1991 dollars). In 1963 the top 1 percent of spenders accounted for 18 percent of costs. Per capita disposable personal income in 1987 was $16,239. In 1963 it was $9,837. Note that the 1987 figure is slightly higher than Berk and Monheit's estimate ($57,000).

3. ERISA encouraged self-insurance by exempting self-insured firms from state health insurance taxes and regulations.

4. For example, 29 percent of companies refused to hire smokers and 6 percent excluded from employment some persons with preexisting health conditions. (Note that these exclusions may be motivated by concerns other than health insurance.)

5. Among those with private insurance coverage, being in poor health meant spending about 2.8 times as much out-of-pocket in 1977 as did those in excellent health, about 4.2 times as much in 1987. There was no similar increase among the uninsured, though. Among this group, out-of-pocket spending in 1977 for those in poor health was also 2.8 times as high as for those in excellent health, but it was only 2.9 times as high in 1987 (Taylor and Banthin 1994).

6. This study did not examine the price of coverage offered to those who inquired.

7. For example, in the Federal Employees' Health Benefits Program, high-risk people chose generous policies and paid considerably more for them than the difference in policy generosity alone could explain (Price and Mays 1985). Much of the difference in risk in these plans may be related to differences in the age of low-cost-plan and high-cost-plan enrollees. As I note below, charging higher prices to younger workers to pay for the costs of coverage of older workers may not be desirable.

8. Long-term health risk contracts avoid many of the problems of multiyear health insurance coverage. Under multiyear coverage, people who move out of the geographic region served by an insurer lose the benefit of their coverage. Furthermore, multiyear-policy holders would have few incentives to economize on their use of health services today, since even those who used services indiscriminately would be protected from future rate hikes under long-term purchase arrangements. For an example of a long-term contract, see Cochrane 1995.

9. Community rating also requires such transfers. The magnitude of the transfers depends on the extent to which adverse selection undoes the effects of community rating.

10. Providers and insurers can recruit healthy populations in a myriad of ingenious ways. They can locate their offices on the second floor of a walkup building; they can move their offices periodically to avoid developing an established, and aging, clientele; they can simply act rudely to their sicker patients or keep them waiting longer.

11. The Clinton health care task force even considered permitting risk rating based on smoking status.

12. My calculations, based on data in Somers and Somers 1961. In a 1957

survey, 39 percent of people over sixty-five had health insurance. In a 1958 survey, spending by all those over sixty-five averaged $177, while spending for all persons averaged $94. Overall, in 1957 those with health insurance spent an average of $106 per person, while those without coverage spent an average of $71 per person. In a 1959 survey, 28 percent of the entire population had no health insurance. In 1959, 9 percent of the population was over sixty-five. I assume that the ratio of spending by the uninsured as opposed to the insured is the same in the elderly and nonelderly population.

13. In 1987 expenditures for personal health spending came to $447 billion, of which people over 65 spent $162 billion. Of the latter sum, Medicare paid $72.2 billion and Medicaid paid $19.5 billion (Waldo et al. 1989).

14. In 1992 Medicare provided $85.3 billion in Part A payments, funded through payroll taxes, and $50.9 billion in Part B claims, funded 75 percent through general revenues and 25 percent through beneficiary premiums (PRO-PAC 1993).

15. Former employers provide almost one-half of the supplementary insurance coverage held by the elderly (ibid.).

16. For women, who typically live longer, Medicare payments exceed contributions by even more.

17. Demographers also expect that post–baby boomers will have fewer children under nineteen to support, a factor that could offset the cost of caring for the elderly.

18. Privately purchased insurance coverage has declined even more steeply. Eligibility expansions in the 1980s, together with the recession of the late 1980s, meant that 3.7 million more people were Medicaid beneficiaries in 1991 than in 1980 (using pre-1988 definitions; Levit, Olin, and Letsch 1992). Part of the decline in private insurance may have occurred in response to the Medicaid expansion. The data for 1980 are from Levit, Olin, and Letsch 1992. Counting changes in the number of uninsured is complex because the working of the questionnaire used for this purpose has changed over time. As many as 5 million extra people may be counted as uninsured using the old definition.

19. My calculations. Hospitals provided $13.4 billion in uncompensated care (CBO 1993c). Estimates for physicians suggest that 9 to 10 percent of billings are uncompensated (Gray 1991; Kilpatrick et al. 1991). Physician billings in 1991 were $142 billion (CBO 1993c). The number of uninsured is from Levit, Olin, and Letsch 1992.

20. Real per capita health spending in 1993 was $3,217 (CBO 1993c). Spending on the uninsured would have to increase by $1,290 per capita to bring them to the national average.

21. In the United States, the scope of rationing differs for the population under sixty-five and the population sixty-five and over. Medicaid beneficiaries

under sixty-five are subject to significant rationing in their care because payments are set at such low levels that in many states, few private doctors will see Medicaid patients. Those not covered by Medicaid are unaffected by its provisions.

Although disparities between Medicare fees and private payments are a continuing concern for Medicare advocates, so far Medicare's fee-based rationing system has had minimal effects on overall service availability for elderly beneficiaries compared with those under sixty-five. Reductions in fees, though, could lead to the development of a two-tier system within Medicare if doctors and hospitals are permitted to charge patients at rates above those the government reimburses (a practice called balance billing). In response to this problem, Medicare has limited payments above the Medicare fee schedule for participating providers. Hospitals serving Medicare patients may not charge Medicare beneficiaries any amount above the public fee schedule and, today, doctors may charge only up to a fixed rate above the schedule.

22. Medicalists might use cost-effectiveness criteria to determine who should be entitled to coverage for a service, but they would not permit those who do not meet cost-effectiveness thresholds to purchase that service, even if they could afford it.

23. The average income of these households was $145,244. There are 96 million households in America (Bureau of the Census 1993b).

24. By contrast, only 9.6 percent of children in the middle third of the income distribution and only 3.8 percent in the lowest third attend private schools (Bureau of the Census 1993b).

25. In Chapter 8 I discuss some recent changes in local school finance intended to reduce these disparities.

26. In fact, by 1977 observers had noted that the actual consumption patterns of the poor had changed appreciably since the minimally adequate bundle was devised (CBO 1977). Food stamp allocations have since been adjusted to reflect the age and sex of recipient families, but do not change as eating habits change (MacDonald 1977).

27. For example, the fraction of all women who have had a pap test at some time in the past three years is higher in the United States than in Canada, even among women with no more than a high-school education (OTA 1993b).

28. According to Serbein (1953), philanthropic contributions amounted to $82 million in 1929 ($479 million in 1991 dollars) and $300 million in 1947 ($1.35 billion in 1991 dollars), an amount 2.8 times as high. By contrast, real national health expenditures increased only 2.1 times over this period.

29. These estimates are unadjusted for differences between the characteristics of the uninsured and the insured.

30. A study of recipients of heart and liver transplants, for example, found

no effect of income on the probability of receiving a transplant and that high-income heart transplant candidates did not jump the queue in front of lower-income candidates (Friedman, Ozminkowksi, and Taylor 1992). Similarly, many hospitals provide heart transplant services to patients who cannot pay (GAO 1989b).

31. The state of Oregon, which rations health care in its Medicaid program by limiting particular services, has established a list of procedures that it will cover and a list of those it will not cover under its public program. For example, Oregon will not fund cancer care for patients with less than a 5 percent chance of survival. The Oregon model appears to separate the decisions of the privately insured from those of the publicly insured. It remains to be seen, though, whether the trade-offs will hold. Doctors are rarely inclined to say a patient has less than a 5 percent chance of survival, and given medical uncertainty, their judgments can hardly be questioned.

32. Between 1975 and 1991, total real cash payments to AFDC families remained constant while total medical payments doubled. On a per-family basis, between 1975 and 1991, AFDC spending fell by one-third, while Medicaid spending rose by one-third (House Ways and Means 1992).

6. The Institutional Structure of Reform

1. The continual revamping of health care systems in other countries suggests that this problem has not been solved satisfactorily anywhere else either.

2. The Canadian model permits variations in the scope and financing of benefits across the provinces and allows each province to control its own health care system.

3. Between 1970 and 1980, real per capita costs in Canada rose at a rate of 3.7 percent per year while costs in the United States rose 4.2 percent per year. Between 1980 and 1990, real per capita costs in Canada rose 4.3 percent per year while costs in the United States rose 4.4 percent per year (OECD 1993b, inflation-adjusted using GDP deflator).

4. Under current financing rules, provinces bear the full burden of rising costs. While almost all U.S. states must balance their budgets, Canadian provinces may run deficits.

5. The U.S. federal deficit amounted to about $1,000 a person in 1993.

6. Real per capita costs, measured in U.S. dollars, increased 7 percent over this period (CBO 1993c).

7. Medicare fee cuts have typically been accompanied by increases in the volume of services provided sufficient to offset about half the revenue effect of the fee cut (Christensen 1992).

8. Medicare regulatory decisions must follow the rule-making process of the Administrative Procedures Act (Buto 1994).

9. In 1980 Medicare and Medicaid paid for 55 percent of the use of intermittent positive pressure breathing. By 1987 these programs were paying for more than 65 percent of a much lower level of use (Duffy and Farley 1993).

10. These figures overstate the extent of the Medicare premium increase. Most of the increase (87 percent of the $54 billion in increased premiums) came from holding Medicare Part B premiums constant as a share of Medicare spending rather than permitting them to drop.

11. As of December 1995, "any willing provider" laws, which mandate that HMOs contract with all willing physicians, had been enacted in Washington, Idaho, Wyoming, Colorado, Illinois, Indiana, Kentucky, Virginia, and Alaska. Patient protection acts, which place somewhat fewer constraints on providers, had been passed in California, Mississippi, Virginia, and Maryland.

12. Some conservative groups do not like the voucher plan either, because it contains an implicit tax hike on higher-income families.

13. The regulations require that Part A deductibles and coinsurance and all Part B coinsurance after payment of the $100 deductible be covered by the Medigap policy (PROPAC 1993).

14. The form of the government's moral-hazard-inducing subsidy in the Medicare market is different, and probably worse, than the employer-based tax subsidy. While the employer-based tax subsidy encourages the purchase of any additional insurance, including insurance that substitutes for public coverage, the Medigap subsidy only encourages the purchase of policies that provide coverage complementary to Medicare. If basic coverage is subsidized, the existence of unregulated supplementation will drive up subsidy costs and reduce the efficiency of the market.

15. In today's private market, people do buy supplemental coverage. Employers often do not pay rebates to workers who obtain coverage from a spouse's employer. By obtaining coverage from both employers, dual-earner families effectively supplement the private coverage they buy (Schur and Taylor 1991).

16. The availability of supplementation acts as a check on the maximum deductible that could be included in a standard plan.

17. Furthermore, in the Health Security Act, payments for supplementation would be exempt from tax.

18. One early discussion of the health care task force centered on developing a new name for the HIPC. A new name was needed to establish the independence of the president's plan from traditional Enthovenian managed competition. The term *health insurance purchasing cooperative* failed on two further fronts. On one hand, *cooperative* was viewed as vaguely "socialist" in tone. *Insurance purchasing,* though, seemed sure to alienate liberals, who felt the plan should bypass insurance altogether. *Health alliance,* the Clinton plan-

ners' replacement, had many virtues. It encompassed both the financing of care and the outcome—health—itself. The term *alliance* sounded dynamic. A consumer cooperative pits consumers against producers, but an alliance allows them all to work together.

19. The Federal Employees' Health Benefit Program (FEHBP) operates in a HIPC-like way. The FEHBP is not a true HIPC, however, because it has paid a (capped) share of the premium of the employee's health plan, not a flat contribution regardless of the plan chosen.

20. One exception, the Memphis Business Group on Health, is a group of 11 large employers in Memphis, Tennessee.

21. Note that states already regulate the solvency, but not the quality, of insurers.

22. See Tallon and Brown 1994 for a discussion of the problems of establishing HIPCs.

23. Integrated systems that combine insurance with service provision might be particularly successful in persuading legislators to enact cost-increasing regulations that favor the insurers' interests.

7. Making Health Policy

1. The actual Clinton plan is much more complicated than this. For example, large regional employers, those with more than 5,000 workers, need not participate in the health alliance.

2. The BNA listing includes some 30 outside consultants. Government rules requiring open meetings made it particularly difficult to bring outside experts into the task force.

3. When programs like Medicare are funded through trust funds, civil servants must develop long-term projections of their costs.

4. Most of the other government employees on the task force came from the Departments of Veterans Affairs and Defense, and, for the most part (although with notable exceptions), were chiefly interested in maintaining the integrity—and funding—of their existing programs.

5. The main program run through the Department of Health and Human Services is Medicare. Within the federal government, Medicare is the largest single regulatory program, far more centralized than many other countries' health system models (including those of Germany and Canada); programs, data, eligibility, payments, and policy are all controlled from Washington. From a regulatory standpoint, the Medicare program is tidy and efficient. Voluminous quantities of data are collected and the effect of every change in the program is carefully monitored.

This flow of information and analysis has made Medicare a model health care bureaucracy. The program boasts a very smart staff with a track record of successfully implementing many administrative innovations. The system of prospective payment by diagnosis-related group was perfected and disseminated through the program. The resource-based relative value scale was developed under contract to the Health Care Financing Administration, the agency that administers Medicare. The administrative costs of running Medicare are lower than the costs of running the Canadian health care system (Etheredge 1992). Medicare bureaucrats are justifiably proud of their program. Orienting health reform toward an expansion of the Medicare system would both extend their power as bureaucrats and reward the expertise that has been developed in the program.

Although the president's plan envisioned a system of competing health insurance companies, few people in the Department of Health and Human Services were sympathetic to this tack. During the early months of the task force process, some Medicare bureaucrats even developed a crafty alternative to the managed-competition plan. They proposed that a plan administered through Medicare be included as a choice available within each health alliance. Medicare bureaucrats would set the premiums and payment rates for this plan. In this way Medicare could take over the entire U.S. health care system, all the while appearing to participate in "managed competition." The Medicare takeover plan was developed at least half in jest and never seemed likely to be incorporated into any final proposal.

6. According to the Congressional Budget Office, a 5 percent VAT on a narrow base (excluding food, medical care, etc.) would raise $51 billion in 1996, while a 5 percent VAT on a broad base would raise $96 billion (CBO 1994b).

7. The president was particularly reluctant to hit high-income taxpayers again after raising the marginal income tax rates on this group to balance the budget. He noted that high health care costs could not be blamed on high-income taxpayers, so it would be difficult to rationalize making them pay the burden of reform.

8. No major industrialized country has a binding global budget on health care that encompasses all health care spending.

9. Of course, with a generous budget and the hybrid financing system discussed above, the plan would have reverted to a medicalist structure soon anyway.

8. Financing Health Care

1. In similar fashion, many elite private colleges today fund their financial-aid packages for poor students by raising tuition to those who pay full price.

In some colleges more than one-third of the cost of tuition goes toward financial aid (Goldin 1995).

2. As early as 1929, 13.6 percent of health care in the United States was publicly funded (Department of Commerce 1975).

3. For example, higher tax rates will deter some people from working more hours and thus reduce the size of the economy.

4. Consider a hypothetical country that contains 80 people who earn $30,000 a year and 20 who earn only $5,000 a year. Suppose, initially, that the higher-income group spends 5 percent of its income on health care, an average of $1,500 each, while the low-income group averages $500 a year (10 percent of income) on self-purchased care. If this society decides that an appropriately equitable distribution of health services would provide the poor half as much care as the rich receive, the average poor person would have to receive $250 more care. This sum could be financed through a 0.2 percent tax on the incomes of higher-income tax payers. Now, though, suppose that a new medical innovation is introduced that prompts higher-income people to double their health spending and lower-income people to increase spending by $40. In order to restore the same level of equity in the distribution of health resources, transfers to the poor would have to be increased to $960, necessitating a quadrupling of the income tax rate to 0.8 percent.

5. Brody et al. (1991) found that 69 percent of physicians in federal public hospitals and 47 percent of physicians in nonfederal public hospitals used streptokinase rather than t-PA. Since about 15 percent of all public hospitals are federal hospitals, this suggests that the weighted average of streptokinase use in public hospitals is 50 percent. Lessler and Avins (1992) found that among the 79 percent of physicians who primarily were using t-PA, 36 percent would switch to streptokinase for a self-pay patient and 27 percent would switch for a Medicaid patient. Physicians who primarily used streptokinase were heavily concentrated in health maintenance organizations.

6. The amount by which they were made worse off depends on the extent to which they *believed* t-PA was a superior drug, not necessarily the actual differential in quality.

7. Many people do complain about "cost shifting" in today's health care market. Privately insured patients complain that reductions in prices paid by the government for health services mean higher prices for them. Employees of large firms assert that they pay higher costs to cover uninsured workers in smaller firms. Actually, in today's health care market, it is unlikely that either outcome occurs. Competing firms, insurers, doctors, and hospitals will almost certainly eliminate the possibility of such "dynamic" cost shifting (see the discussion in Morrissey 1994). Nonetheless, these complaints imply not so much that cost shifting itself is inappropriate than that the burden of caring for the poor is unevenly allocated so that not everyone is paying a fair share.

8. For example, the chairman of MCI communications, William Mc-Gowan, donated $1 million to the hospital where he had undergone a heart transplant operation (Brown et al. 1990). A philanthropist in Gross Pointe, Michigan, who later died of cancer, donated $3 million for treatment of the disease to a Detroit hospital ("Hospital Benefactor" 1989). A physician in Washington, D.C., made a small donation to a fund-raising campaign for the hospital that had saved her life as an infant 33 years earlier (Levey 1994).

9. The demand for health services is relatively inelastic (unresponsive to prices), while the supply of services, especially in the long run, is likely to be relatively elastic (responsive to prices). This means that most of the tax will be borne by patients.

10. A tax on health care also makes sense under a more pragmatic analysis that entirely rejects the externality argument. Empirical estimates suggest that a moderate tax on health care to fund health care for the needy would not cause substantial changes in individual behavior. Estimates from the literature on the tax subsidy to health insurance premiums suggest that entirely removing that subsidy would reduce national health spending by only 5 to 10 percent. This relatively low level of responsiveness suggests that a tax on health spending would not greatly distort national health spending decisions at any given time. Furthermore, the tax rate would be held constant at a low level and, unlike other kinds of taxes used to fund health care, would not increase with increases in health costs. Any distortionary impact of the tax would not increase over time.

11. This 60 percent figure reflects differences in the level of health of the insured and uninsured populations and is based on an estimate that overall spending by the uninsured would increase by 57 percent if they received an average-quality health insurance package (OTA 1994). Actual spending by the uninsured is closer to 50 percent of average spending, because the uninsured tend to be younger and healthier than average.

12. The tax rate needed to correct for the externality is $x \cdot y/(1-y)$, where x is the relative size of the minimally adequate bundle (e.g., 60 percent) and y is the proportion of the population of concern (e.g., ⅓). If the minimally adequate bundle were defined at 50 percent of the average and the population of concern was the bottom ¼ of the population, the tax rate would be only 17 percent.

13. Approximately half of all seniors have incomes below two times the poverty line (DHHS 1995). Note that this calculation assumes that coverage for the Medicare elderly would continue at the current level, rather than at 60 percent of the average level.

14. The tax would have to fund $115 billion in Medicaid expenditures and about $42 billion in spending for the 23 million uninsured with incomes below twice the poverty level, assuming that average spending by the uninsured

would be equal to average spending by low-income adults in the Medicaid program (DHHS 1995).

15. The availability of private insurance for services in the private sector might lead to an increased call on public-sector resources (as is the case for Medicare supplemental coverage). This increased usage would be relatively small, because the public sector in a single-payer system does not require co-payments and deductibles. It might, however, be appropriate to add a further tax on private health insurance coverage.

16. This calculation assumes initial spending of $4,000 per capita, 3 percent per capita spending growth in the tax-financed system, and 6 percent per capita spending growth in the private system. My analysis assumes that the private sector provides supplemental care and does not divert care from the public sector. If the private sector diverted care from the public sector, per capita spending in the public sector would grow faster.

References

Abbreviations

AEI	American Enterprise Institute
AHA	American Hospital Association
AMA	American Medical Association
BNA	Bureau of National Affairs
CBO	Congressional Budget Office
CEA	Council of Economic Advisers
CRS	Congressional Research Service
DHHS	Department of Health and Human Services
EBRI	Employee Benefits Research Institute
GAO	General Accounting Office
GHAA	Group Health Association of America
HCFR	*Health Care Financing Review*
HIAA	Health Insurance Association of America
JAMA	*Journal of the American Medical Association*
JAVMA	*Journal of the American Veterinary Medicine Association*
NBER	National Bureau of Economic Research
NEJM	*New England Journal of Medicine*
OECD	Organization for Economic Cooperation and Development
OMB	Office of Management and Budget
OTA	Office of Technology Assessment
PROPAC	Prospective Payment Assessment Commission

Aaron, Henry J. 1991. *Serious and Unstable Condition: Financing America's Health Care*. Washington, D.C.: Brookings Institution.

———. 1993. "Paying for Health Care." *Domestic Affairs* 2 (Winter 1993/94): 23–78.

Aaron, Henry J. 1994. *Roundtable Discussion on the Economics of Health Care*. Joint Economic Committee. Senate Hearing 103–585 (April). Washington, D.C.: Government Printing Office.

251

Aaron, Henry J., and William B. Schwartz. 1984. *The Painful Prescription: Rationing Hospital Care.* Washington, D.C.: Brookings Institution.

Alpha Center. 1995. "New York May Abandon Rate Setting." *State Initiative's Newsletter,* September/October.

American Board of Medical Specialists. 1991. Fax to author.

American Council of Life Insurers. 1993. *Life Insurance Fact Book Update.* Washington, D.C.: American Council of Life Insurers.

American Hospital Association (AHA). Various years, 1972–1993. *Hospital Statistics.* Chicago: AHA.

American Medical Association (AMA). Various years, 1983–1994. *Socioeconomic Characteristics of Medical Practice.* Edited by Martin L. Gonzalez. Chicago: Center for Health Policy Research.

Anderson, Geoffrey M., Kevin Grumbach, Harold S. Luft, Leslie L. Ross, Cameron Mustard, and Robert Brook. 1993. "Use of Coronary Artery Bypass Surgery in the United States and Canada: Influence of Age and Income." *JAMA* 269 (13; April 7): 1661–1666.

Andreoni, James. 1988. "Privately-Provided Public Goods in a Large Economy: The Limits of Altruism." *Journal of Public Economics* 35l: 57–73.

Arrow, Kenneth J. 1963. "Uncertainty and the Welfare Economics of Medical Care." *American Economic Review* 53 (December): 941–973.

Auerbach, Alan J., Jagadeesh Gokhale, and Laurence J. Kotlikoff. 1993. "Generational Accounts and Lifetime Tax Rates, 1990–91." *Economic Review* (First Quarter 1993): 2–13.

Azevedo, David. 1993. "Canada: The Truth about Queues." *Medical Economics,* May 24: 168–183.

Balz, Dan. 1994. "Health Plan Was Albatross for Democrats." *Washington Post,* November 18, final edition, sec. A, p. 1, col. 1.

Barer, Morris L., Robert G. Evans, and Roberta Labelle. 1985. *The Frozen North: Controlling Physicians' Costs through Controlling Fees—The Canadian Experience* (November). U.S. Office of Technology Assessment Contractor Report. Washington, D.C.: OTA.

Barkin, Martin. 1992. "Ontario's Health Care System at the Crossroads." In *Restructuring Canada's Health System: How Do We Get There from Here?,* edited by Raisa B. Deber and Gail G. Thompson, 3–7. Toronto: University of Toronto Press.

Bartel, Ann P., and Frank R. Lichtenberg. 1987. "The Comparative Advantage of Educated Workers in Implementing New Technology." *Review of Economics and Statistics* 69 (February): 1–11.

Baumgardner, James R. 1991. "The Interaction between Forms of Insurance Contract and Types of Technological Change in Medical Care." *RAND Journal of Economics* 22 (Spring): 36–53.

Baumol, William J. 1967. "Macroeconomics of Unbalanced Growth: The Anatomy of Urban Crisis." *American Economic Review* (June): 415–426.

Beauregard, Karen M. 1991. "Persons Denied Private Health Insurance Due to Poor Health." *National Medical Expenditure Survey.* Data Summary 4. Rockville, Md.: Agency for Health Care Policy and Research.

Becker, Edmund R., and Frank A. Sloan. 1985. "Hospital Ownership and Performance." *Economic Inquiry* 23 (January): 21–36.

Berenson, Robert A. 1994. "Do Physicians Recognize Their Own Best Interests?" *Health Affairs* 13 (2; Spring): 185–193.

Berk, Marc L., and Alan C. Monheit. 1992. "The Concentration of Health Expenditures: An Update." *Health Affairs* 11 (4; Winter): 145–149.

Bernstein, Aaron, and Susan B. Garland. 1990. "Health Care Costs: Trying to Cool the Fever—Making it Pay to Stay Healthy." *Business Week* 3160 (May 21): 46–47.

Best's Life and Health Insurance Reports. 1992. Oldwick, N.J.: A. M. Best.

Blackburn, McKinley L., and David E. Bloom. 1995. *Changes in the Structure of Family Income Inequality in the United States and Other Industrial Nations during the 1980s.* National Bureau of Economic Research Working Paper, no. 4754. Cambridge, Mass.: NBER.

Blendon, Robert J., John Benson, Karen Donelan, Robert Leitman, Humphrey Taylor, Christian Koeck, and David Gitterman. 1995. "Who Has the Best Health Care System? A Second Look." *Health Affairs* 14 (4; Winter): 220–230.

Blendon, Robert J., Karen Donelan, Robert Leitman, and Arnold Epstein. 1993. "Health Reform Lessons Learned from Physicians in Three Nations." *Health Affairs* 12 (3; Fall): 194–203.

Blustein, Janice. 1993. "High-Technology Cardiac Procedures: The Impact of Service Availability on Service Use in New York State." *JAMA* 270 (3; July 21): 344–349.

Boer, Germain. 1994. "Five Modern Myths." *Accountancy* 113 (June): 82–83.

Bovbjerg, Randall R., and Kenneth R. Petronis. 1994. "The Relationship between Physicians' Malpractice Claims History and Later Claims: Does the Past Predict the Future?" *JAMA* 272 (18; November 9): 1421–1426.

Brody, Baruch, Nelda Wary, Sherry Bame, Carol Ashton, Nancy Petersen, and Mary Harward. 1991. "The Impact of Economic Considerations on Clinical Decision Making: The Case of Thrombolytic Therapy." *Medical Care* 29 (9; September): 899–910.

Brook, Robert H., and Elizabeth A. McGlynn. 1994. "Maintaining Quality of Care." In *Health Services Research: Key to Health Policy,* edited by Eli Ginzberg, 284–314. Cambridge, Mass.: Harvard University Press.

Brown, Charles, James Hamilton, and James Medoff. 1990. *Employers Large and Small.* Cambridge, Mass.: Harvard University Press.

Brown, Lawrence D. 1993. "Dogmatic Slumbers: American Business and Health Policy." *Journal of Health Politics, Policy, and Law* 18 (2; Summer): 339–357.

Brown, Randall S., Dolores Gurnick Clement, Jerrold W. Hill, Sheldon M. Retchin, and Jeannette W. Bergeron. 1993. "Do HMOs Work for Medicare?" *HCFR* 15 (1; Fall): 7–23.

Brown, Warren, Cindy Skrzycki, John Burgess, and Karen Swiskin. 1990. "You Gotta Have Heart." *Washington Post,* August 6, sec. F, p. 3, col. 1.

Brownstein, Ronald. 1993. "By 2–1 Margin, Public Backs Health Care Plan." *Los Angeles Times,* September 30, sec. A, p. 1, col. 2.

Bureau of the Census. 1992. *An Aging World II.* International Population Reports. Series P25, 92–93. Washington, D.C.: Government Printing Office.

Bureau of the Census. 1993a. *Money Income of Households, Families, and Persons in the United States, 1992.* Current Population Reports. Series P60-184. Washington, D.C.: Government Printing Office.

Bureau of the Census. 1993b. *School Enrollment—Social and Economic Characteristics of Students: October 1992.* Washington, D.C.: Government Printing Office.

Bureau of National Affairs (BNA). 1993. *Health Care Policy Report,* vol. 1 (March 8).

Burke, Gerald. 1993. "It's Time to Add Cost-Effectiveness to the Healthcare Reform Equation." *Modern Healthcare* 23 (29; July 29): 22.

Burner, Sally T., Daniel R. Waldo, and David R. McKusick. 1992. "National Health Expenditures: Projections through 2030." *HCFR* 14 (1; Fall): 1–29.

Burns, Eveline M. 1973. *Health Services for Tomorrow: Trends and Issues.* New York: Dunellen Publishing.

Buto, Kathleen A. 1994. "How Can Medicare Keep Pace with Cutting-Edge Technology?" *Health Affairs* 13 (3; Summer): 137–140.

Call, Robert S., Thomas F. Smith Thomas, Elsie Morris, Martin D. Chapman, and Thomas A. E. Platts-Mills. 1992. "Risk Factors for Asthma in Inner City Children." *Journal of Pediatrics* 121 (6; December): 862–866.

Canada. Health and Welfare Canada. 1990. *National Health Expenditures in Canada, 1975–87.* Ottawa: Health and Welfare Canada.

Canada Health. 1993. *Canada Health Act Annual Report, 1992–1993.* Ottawa: Health and Welfare Canada.

Carr, Jack, and Frank Mathewson. 1990. "The Economics of Law Firms: A

Study in the Legal Organization of the Firm." *Journal of Law and Economics* 33 (October): 307–330.

Chassin, Mark, Jacqueline Kosecoff, R. E. Park, Contance M. Winslow, Katharine L. Kahn, Nancy J. Merrick, Joan Keesey, Arlene Fink, David H. Solomon, Robert H. Brook. 1987. "Does Inappropriate Use Explain Geographic Variations in the Use of Health Care Services?" *JAMA* 258 (18; November 13): 2533–2537.

Chernick, Howard, Martin Holmer, and Daniel Weinberg. 1987. "Tax Policy toward Health Insurance and the Demand for Medical Services." *Journal of Health Economics* 6 (1; March): 1–25.

Christensen, Sandra. 1992. "Volume Responses to Exogenous Changes in Medicare's Payment Policies." *Health Services Research* 27 (1; April): 65–79.

Christensen, Sandra, Stephen H. Long, and Jack Rodgers. 1987. "Acute Health Care Costs for the Aged Medicare Population: Overview and Policy Options." *Milbank Quarterly* 65 (3): 397–425.

Clymer, Adam. 1993. "Hillary Clinton Accuses Insurers of Lying about Health Proposal." *New York Times*, November 2, late edition, sec. A, p. 1, col. 1.

Cochrane, John H. 1995. "Time-Consistent Health Insurance." *Journal of Political Economy* 103 (3; June): 445–473.

Coffey, Rosanna M. 1983. *Patients in Public General Hospitals: Who Pays, How Sick?* HCUP [Hospital Cost and Utilization Project] Research Note 2 (September). Rockville, Md.: National Center for Health Services Research.

Committee on the Costs of Medical Care. 1932. *Medical Care for the American People: The Final Report*. Chicago: University of Chicago Press.

Congressional Budget Office (CBO). 1977. *The Food Stamp Program: Income or Food Supplementation* (January). Washington, D.C.: Government Printing Office.

———. 1979. *Profile of Health Care Coverage: The Haves and Have Nots* (March). Washington, D.C.: Government Printing Office.

———. 1992. *Economic Implications of Rising Health Care Costs* (October). Washington, D.C.: Government Printing Office.

———. 1993a. *Baby Boomers in Retirement: An Early Perspective* (September). Washington, D.C.: Government Printing Office.

———. 1993b. *Estimates of Health Care Proposals from the 102nd Congress* (July). Washington, D.C.: Government Printing Office.

———. 1993c. *Trends in Health Spending: An Update* (June). Washington, D.C.: Government Printing Office.

———. 1994a. *Economic and Budget Outlook: Fiscal Years 1995–1999* (February). Washington, D.C.: Government Printing Office.

———. 1994b. *Reducing the Deficit: Spending and Revenue Options* (March). Washington, D.C.: Government Printing Office.

———. 1994c. *Reducing Entitlement Spending* (September). Washington, D.C.: Government Printing Office.

———. 1994d. *The Tax Treatment of Employment-Based Health Insurance* (March). Washington, D.C.: Government Printing Office.

———. 1995. *Cost Estimate: Medicare Reconciliation Language Reported by the Senate Committee on Finance on October 17, 1995* (October). Washington, D.C.: CBO.

Congressional Research Service (CRS). 1988. *Health Insurance and the Uninsured: Background Data and Analysis.* Washington, D.C.: Government Printing Office.

Cooper, Philip F., and Ayah E. Johnson. 1993. *Employment-Related Health Insurance in 1987.* National Medical Expenditure Survey Research Findings 17. Rockville, Md.: Agency for Health Care Policy and Research.

Council of Economic Advisers (CEA). Various years, 1990–1995. *Economic Report of the President.* Washington, D.C.: Government Printing Office.

Cowan, Cathy A., and Patricia A. McDonnell. 1993. "Business, Households, and Governments: Health Spending 1991." *HCFR* 14 (3; Spring): 227–249.

Coyte, Peter C., James G. Wright, Gillian A. Hawker, Claire Bombardier, Robert S. Dittus, John E. Paul, Deborah A. Freund, and Elsa Ho. 1994. "Waiting Times for Knee-Replacement Surgery in the United States and Ontario." *NEJM* 331 (16; October 20): 1068–1071.

Crittenden, Robert A. 1993. "State Model: Washington—Managed Competition and Premium Caps in Washington State." *Health Affairs* 12 (2; Summer): 82–88.

Cutler, David M. 1994. "A Guide to Health Care Reform." *Journal of Economic Perspectives* 8 (3; Summer): 13–29.

Danzon, Patricia, Mark Pauly, and Raynard S. Kington. 1990. "The Effects of Malpractice Litigation on Physicians' Fees and Incomes." *American Economic Review* 80 (May): 122–127.

Danzon, Patricia M. 1985. *Medical Malpractice: Theory, Evidence, and Public Policy.* Cambridge: Harvard University Press.

———. 1992. "Hidden Overhead Costs: Is Canada's System less Expensive?" *Health Affairs* 11 (1; Spring): 21–43.

De Lew, Nancy, George Greenberg, and Kraig Kinchen. 1992. "A Layman's Guide to the U.S. Health Care System." *HCFR* 14 (1; Fall): 151–169.

Department of Commerce. 1975. *Historical Statistics of the United States: Colonial Times to 1970*. Washington, D.C.: Government Printing Office.

———. Various years, 1980–1993. *Current Population Survey* (data tapes). Washington, D.C.

———. 1993. *State and Metropolitan Area Data Book*. Washington, D.C.: Government Printing Office.

Department of Health and Human Services (DHHS). Various years, 1980–1995. *Health, U.S.* Washington, D.C.: Government Printing Office.

Department of Labor. Various years, 1986–1993. *Consumer Expenditure Survey*. Washington, D.C.: Government Printing Office.

— ——. Bureau of Labor Statistics. 1991a. *Employee Benefits in Medium and Large Private Establishments*. Washington, D.C.: Government Printing Office.

———. 1991b. "International Comparisons of Manufacturing Productivity and Unit Labor Cost Trends." *U.S. Department of Labor Bulletin* (December 2): 92–752.

Department of Transportation. National Highway Traffic Safety Administration. 1991. *Highway Safety*. Washington, D.C.: Government Printing Office.

DeWitt, Paula Mergenhagen. 1993. "In Pursuit of Pregnancy." *American Demographics* 15 (May): 48–53.

Diehl, Andrew K. 1993. "Laparoscopic Cholecystectomy: Too Much of a Good Thing?" *JAMA* 270 (12; September 22): 1469–1470.

Donabedian, Avedis. 1984. "Volume, Quality, and the Regionalization of Health Care Services." *Medical Care* 22 (2; February): 95–97.

Dougherty, Charles J. 1988. *American Health Care: Realities, Rights, and Reforms*. New York: Oxford University Press.

Drew, Elizabeth. 1994. *On the Edge: The Clinton Presidency*. New York: Simon and Schuster.

Duffy, John. 1993. *From Humors to Medical Science*. 2d ed. Chicago: University of Illinois Press.

Duffy, Sarah Q., and Dean E. Farley. 1993. *Intermittent Positive Pressure Breathing: Old Technologies Rarely Die*. Division of Provider Studies Research Note 17. Rockville, Md.: Agency for Health Care Policy and Research.

Dynan, Linda Marie. 1994. "The Organization of Medical Practice." Ph.D. dissertation, Columbia University.

Eddy, David M., and John Billings. 1988. "The Quality of Medical Evidence: Implications for Quality of Care." *Health Affairs* 7 (1; Spring): 19–32.

Eddy, David M. 1984. "Variations in Physician Practice: The Role of Uncertainty." *Health Affairs* 3 (2; Summer): 74–89.

Elitzak, Howard. 1992. "Marketing Bill Is the Largest Chunk of Food Expenditures." *Food Review* 15 (July–September): 12–15.

Employee Benefits Research Institute (EBRI). 1993. *Sources of Health Insurance and Characteristics of the Uninsured.* Issue Brief no. 133. Washington, D.C.: EBRI.

———. 1995. *Sources of Health Insurance and Characteristics of the Uninsured.* Issue Brief no. 158. Washington, D.C.: EBRI.

Enthoven, Alain. 1993. "Why Managed Care Has Failed to Contain Health Costs." *Health Affairs* 12 (3; Fall): 27–43.

Escarce, Jose J. 1993. "Would Eliminating Differences in Physician Practice Style Reduce Geographic Variations in Cataract Surgery Rates?" *Medical Care* 31 (12; December): 1106–1118.

Etheredge, Lynn. 1992. "Management Options for Health System Reform: Policy Choices and Administrative Costs." Paper presented at Conference on Administrative Costs in the U.S. Health Care System (February).

Evans, Robert G. 1974. "Supplier-Induced Demand: Some Empirical Evidence and Implications." In *The Economics of Health and Medical Care,* edited by Mark Perlman, 162–173. London: Macmillan.

Evans, Robert G., Jonathan Lomas, Morris L. Barer, Roberta J. Labelle, Catherine Fooks, Gregory L. Stoddart, Geoffrey M. Anderson, David Feeny, Amiram Gafni, George W. Torrance, and William G. Tholl. 1989. "Controlling Health Expenditures—The Canadian Reality." *NEJM* 320 (9; March 2): 571–577.

Fallows, James. 1995. "Public Affairs: A Triumph of Misinformation." *Atlantic Monthly,* January: 26–37.

Farley, Pamela A. 1986. *Private Health Insurance in the United States.* National Health Care Expenditures Study Data Preview 23 (September). Rockville, Md.: DHHS, National Center for Health Services Research.

Fein, Rashi. 1986. *Medical Care, Medical Costs.* Cambridge: Harvard University Press.

Feldman, Roger, and Bryan Dowd. 1991. "A New Estimate of the Welfare Loss of Excess Health Insurance." *American Economic Review* 81 (March): 297–301.

Feldstein, Martin S. 1973. "The Welfare Loss of Excess Health Insurance." *Journal of Political Economy* 81 (2, pt. 2; March): 251–280.

———. 1977. "Quality Change and the Demand for Hospital Care." *Econometrica* 45 (7; October): 1681–1702.

Feldstein, Paul J. 1988. *Health Care Economics.* 3d ed. New York: Wiley.

Flood, Ann Barry, W. Richard Scott, and Wayne Ewy. 1984. "Does Practice Make Perfect?" *Medical Care* 22 (2; February): 98–125.

Folland, Sherman, Allen C. Goodman, and Miron Stano. 1993. *The Economics of Health and Health Care.* New York: Macmillan.

Follmann, J. F. 1963. *Medical Care and Health Insurance.* Homewood, Ill.: R. D. Irwin.

Fossett, James W. 1994. "Cost Containment and Rate Setting." In *Making Health Reform Work: The View from the States,* edited by John J. DiIullio, Jr., and Richard R. Nathan. Washington, D.C.: Brookings Institution.

Frech, H. E., III. 1985. "The Property Rights Theory of the Firm: Some Evidence from the U.S. Nursing Home Industry." *Zeitschrift fur Staatswissenschaft* 141:146–166.

Friedman, Bernard, Ronald J. Ozminkowski, and Zachary Taylor. 1992. "Excess Demand and Patient Selection for Heart and Liver Transplantation." In *Health Economics Worldwide,* edited by Peter Zweifel and H. E. Frech III, 161–186. Dordrecht, Netherlands: Kluwer Academic Publishers.

Friedman, Milton, and Simon Kuznets. 1945. *Income from Independent Professional Practices.* National Bureau of Economic Research General Series, no. 45. New York: NBER.

Friedman, Thomas L. 1992. "Clinton Economic Session Yields Clear Goals, but Solutions Clash." *New York Times,* December 16, late edition, sec. A, p. 1, col. 2.

Frum, David. 1994. *Dead Right.* New York: Basic Books.

Fuchs, Victor. 1974. *Who Shall Live?* New York: Basic Books.

———. 1986. *The Health Economy.* Cambridge: Harvard University Press.

———. 1994a. "The Clinton Plan: A Researcher Examines Reform." *Health Affairs* 13 (1; Spring): 102–114.

———. 1994b. "A Conversation about Health Care Reform." *Western Journal of Medicine* 161 (1; July): 83–86.

———. 1994c. "Health System Reform: A Different Approach." *JAMA* 272 (7; August 17): 560–563.

Gabel, Jon, Roger Formisano, Barbara Lohr, and Steven Di Carlo. 1991. "Tracing the Cycle of Health Insurance." *Health Affairs* 10 (4; Winter): 48–61.

Gabel, Jon, Derek Liston, Gail Jensen, and Jill Marsteller. 1994. "The Health Insurance Picture in 1993: Some Rare Good News," *Health Affairs* 13 (1; Spring): 327–336.

Gallup Poll. Various years, 1937–1995. Wilmington, Del.: Scholarly Resources.

Galt, Alan. 1994. *Regulation, Deregulation, Reregulation: The Future of the Banking, Insurance, and Securities Industries.* New York: John Wiley.

Gaumer, Gary L. 1984. "Regulating Health Professionals: A Review of the

Empirical Literature." *Milbank Memorial Fund Quarterly* 62 (3): 380–416.

General Accounting Office (GAO). 1986. *Tax Policy: Information on the Stock and Mutual Segments of the Life Insurance Industry.* Washington, D.C.: GAO.

———. 1987. *Medicare and Medicaid: Effects of Recent Legislation on Program and Beneficiary Costs.* Washington, D.C.: GAO.

———. 1989a. *Heart Transplant Issues.* Washington, D.C.: GAO.

———. 1989b. *International Trade: The Health of the U.S. Steel Industry.* Washington, D.C.: GAO.

———. 1991. *Canadian Health Insurance: Lessons for the United States.* Washington, D.C.: GAO.

———. 1992a. *Access to Health Insurance: State Efforts to Assist Small Businesses.* Washington, D.C.: GAO.

———. 1992b. *Canadian Health Insurance: Estimated Costs and Savings for the United States.* Washington, D.C.: GAO.

———. 1992c. *Health Insurance: Vulnerable Payers Lose Billions to Fraud and Abuse.* Washington, D.C.: GAO.

———. 1993a. *Medicaid Data Improvements Needed to Help Manage Health Care Program.* Washington, D.C.: GAO.

———. 1993b. *1993 German Health Reforms New Cost Control Initiatives: Report to the Chairman, Committee on Governmental Affairs, U.S. Senate.* Washington, D.C.: GAO.

———. 1993c. *Utilization Review Information on External Review Organizations: Fact Sheet for the Chairman, Select Committee on Aging, U.S. House of Representatives.* Washington, D.C.: GAO.

Gentry, Dwight L., and William A. Hailey. 1980. "The CEO: Beginnings and Backgrounds." *Business* 30 (September/October): 15–19.

Gertler, Paul J. 1989. "Subsidies, Quality, and the Regulation of Nursing Homes." *Journal of Public Economics* 38: 33–52.

Getzen, Thomas E. 1984. "A 'Brand Name Firm' Theory of Medical Group Practice." *Journal of Industrial Economics* 33 (December): 199–215.

Ginzberg, Eli, and Miriam Ostow. 1994. *The Road to Reform.* New York: Free Press.

Glied, Sherry. 1993. "Canadian Healthcare: Fact, Fiction, and Fantasy." Unpublished manuscript.

———. 1994. *Revising the Tax Treatment of Employer-Provided Health Insurance.* Washington, D.C.: AEI Press.

Goddeeris, John H. 1984. "Medical Insurance, Technological Change, and Welfare." *Economic Inquiry* 22 (January): 56–67.

Goldblatt, Peter. 1989. "Mortality by Social Class, 1971–1985." *Population Trends* 56 (Summer).

Goldin, Davidson. 1995. "Increasingly, Those Paying Full Tuition Aid Poorer Peers." *New York Times,* March 22, late edition, Sec. B, p. 7, col. 1.

Gornick, Marian, Alma McMillan, and James Lubitz. 1993. "A Longitudinal Perspective on Patterns of Medicare Payments." *Health Affairs* 12 (2; Summer): 140–150.

Graig, Laurene A. 1993. *Health of Nations: An International Perspective on U.S. Health Care Reform.* Washington, D.C.: Congressional Quarterly.

Gray, Bradford H. 1991. *The Profit Motive and Patient Care: The Changing Accountability of Doctors and Hospitals.* Cambridge: Harvard University Press.

Greenfield, Sheldon, Eugene, C. Nelson, Michael Zubkoff, Willard Manning, William Rogers, Richard L. Kravitz, Adam Keller, Alan R. Tarlov, and John E. Ware. 1992. "Variations in Resource Utilization among Medical Specialties and Systems of Care." *JAMA* 267 (12; March 25): 1624–1630.

Greenhouse, Steven. 1992. "Clinton's Aides Seek Bigger Cut in Deficit Early." *New York Times.* December 19, late edition, sec. A, p. 8, col. 6.

Group Health Association of America (GHAA). *National Directory of HMOs.* Washington, D.C.: GHAA.

Grumbach, Kevin, and Philip R. Lee. 1991. "How Many Physicians Can We Afford?" *JAMA* 265 (18; May 8): 2369–2372.

Havighurst, Clark C. 1990. "The Professional Paradigm of Medical Care: Obstacle to Decentralization." *Jurimetrics Journal* 30 (Summer): 415–430.

Hayek, Friedrich A. 1945. "The Use of Knowledge in Society." *American Economic Review* 35 (September): 519–530.

Hayes, James A., Joseph B. Cole, and David I. Meisleman. 1993. "Health Insurance Derivatives: The Newest Application of Modern Financial Risk Management." *Business Economics* 28 (April): 36–40.

Health Care Task Force. 1993. Background material.

Health Coverage Availability and Affordability Act of 1996. Public Law 104–191. Washington, D.C.: Government Printing Office.

Health Insurance Association of America (HIAA). 1992. *Source Book of Health Insurance Data, 1991.* Washington, D.C.: HIAA.

———. 1993. *Source Book of Health Insurance Data, 1992.* Washington, D.C.: HIAA.

Health Security Act. 1993. Washington, D.C.: Government Printing Office.

Healy, William L., and David Finn. 1994. "The Hospital Cost and the Cost of the Implant for Total Knee Arthroplasty: A Comparison between 1983 and 1991 for One Hospital." *Journal of Bone and Joint Surgery* 76 (6; June): 801–806.

Heller, Peter S., Richard Hemming, and Peter W. Kohnert. 1986. *Aging and Social Expenditures in the Major Industrialized Countries: 1980–2025.* Washington, D.C.: International Monetary Fund.

Hilborne, Lee H., Lucian L. Leape, James P. Kahan, Rolla Edward Park, Caren J. Kamberg, and Robert H. Brook. 1991. *Percutaneous Transluminal Coronary Angioplasty: A Literature Review and Ratings of Appropriateness and Necessity.* Santa Monica, Calif.: RAND.

Himmelstein, David U., and Steffie Woolhandler. 1988. "The Corporate Compromise: A Marxist View of Health Maintenance Organizations and Prospective Payment" *Annals of Internal Medicine* 109 (6; September): 494–501.

———. 1989. "A National Health Program for the United States: A Physician's Proposal." *NEJM* 320 (2; January 12): 102–108.

Hoffmeyer, Ulrich K., and Thomas R. McCarthy. 1994. *Financing Health Care,* vol. 1. Dordrecht, Netherlands: Kluwer Academic Publishers.

Holahan, John, Diane Rowland, Judith Feder, and D. Helsam. 1993. "Explaining the Recent Growth in Medicaid Spending." *Health Affairs* 12 (3; Fall): 177–193.

Hood, Ann Barry, W. Richard Scott, and Wayne Evoy. 1984. "Does Practice Make Perfect? Part I." *Medical Care* 22 (2; February): 98–114.

"Hospital Benefactor Wertz Dies 3 Days after Bequest." 1989. *Detroit News,* August 22, sec. D, p. 1, col. 5.

House Committee on the Budget Republican Staff. 1992. "Redefining AIDS: Its Impact on Health and Disability Entitlement Spending." *Republican Staff Report* (November 30).

House Ways and Means Committee. Various years, 1981–1994. *Green Book.* Washington, D.C.: Government Printing Office.

Iacocca, Lee. 1988. *Talking Straight.* New York: Bantam Books.

ICF Incorporated. 1987. *Health Care Coverage and Costs in Small and Large Businesses.* Report prepared for the Office of Advocacy. Small Business Administration. Washington, D.C.

Inlander, Charles B., Lowell S. Levin, and Ed Weiner. 1988. *Medicine on Trial: The Appalling Story of Medical Ineptitude and the Arrogance That Overlooks It.* New York: Pantheon Books.

Institute of Medicine. 1985. *Assessing Medical Technologies: Report of a Study.* Washington, D.C.: National Academy Press.

———. 1995. *The Nation's Physician Workforce: Options for Balancing Supply and Requirements.* Edited by Kathleen N. Lohr, Neal A. Vanselow, and Don E. Detmer. Washington, D.C.: Institute of Medicine.

Insurance Information Institute. 1990. *Property and Casualty Insurance Facts.* New York: Insurance Information Institute.

Jacobs, Lawrence R., and Robert Y. Shapiro. 1993. "The Duality of Public Opinion: Personal Interests and the National Interest in Health Care Reform." *Domestic Affairs* 2 (Winter 1993/94): 245–259.

Jacobs, Lawrence R., Robert Y. Shapiro, and Eli C. Schulman. 1993. "Medical Care in the United States—an Update." *Public Opinion Quarterly* 57 (3): 394–427.

Juhn, Chin-hui, Kevin Murphy, and Brooks Pierce. 1993. "Wage Inequality and the Rise in Returns to Skill." *Journal of Political Economy* 101 (3; June): 410–442.

Kasper, J. F., A. G. Mulley, and J. F. Wennberg. 1992. "Developing Shared Decision-Making Programs to Improve the Quality of Health Care." *QRB: Quality Review Bulletin* 18 (6; June): 182.

Katz, Lawrence, Gary Loveman, and David Blanchflower. 1993. *A Comparison of Changes in the Structure of Wages in Four OECD Countries.* NBER Working Paper no. 4297. Cambridge, Mass.: NBER.

Kessel, Reuben. 1958. "Price Discrimination in Medicine." *Journal of Law and Economics* 1 (October): 25.

Khandker, Rezaul K., and Willard G. Manning. 1992. "The Impact of Utilization Review on Costs and Utilization." In *Health Economics Worldwide,* edited by Peter Zweifel and H. E. Frech III, 47–62. Dordrecht, Netherlands: Kluwer Academic Publishers.

Kilpatrick, Kerry E., Michael K. Miller, Jeffrey W. Dwyer, and Dan Nissen. 1991. "Uncompensated Care Provided by Private Practice Physicians in Florida." *Health Services Research* 26 (3; August): 277–302.

Kindig, David A., James M. Cultice, and Fitzhugh Mullan. 1993. "The Elusive Generalist Physician: Can We Reach a 50% Goal?" *JAMA* 270 (9; September): 1069–1073.

Kissick, William L. 1994. *Medicine's Dilemmas: Infinite Needs versus Finite Resources.* New Haven: Yale University Press.

Klein, Benjamin, and Keith Leffler. 1981. "The Role of Market Forces in Assuring Quality." *Journal of Political Economy* 89 (4; August): 615–641.

Kronick, Richard. 1993. "Where Should the Buck Stop: Federal and State Responsibilities in Health Care Financing Reform." *Health Affairs* 12 (Supplement): 87–98.

———. 1994. "Redistributing Health Care Resources without Redistributing Income." *Journal of Health Politics, Policy, and Law* 19 (3; Fall): 543–553.

"Lawyers' Bottom Line." 1993. Survey of Law Firm Economics, Altma Weil

Pensa Publications, reproduced in the *Wall Street Journal,* July 15, sec. B, p. 6.

Leape, Lucian L. 1989. "Unnecessary Surgery." *Health Services Research* 24 (3; August): 351–407.

Leape, Lucian L., Lee H. Hilborne, James P. Kahan, William B. Stason, Rolla Edward Park, Caren J. Kamberg, and Robert H. Brook. 1991. *Coronary Artery Bypass Graft: A Literature Review and Ratings of Appropriateness and Necessity.* Santa Monica, Calif.: RAND.

Lefkowitz, Doris C., and Alan C. Monheit. 1991. "Health Insurance, Use of Health Services, and Health Care Expenditures." *National Medical Expenditure Survey Research Findings* 12. Rockville, Md.: Agency for Health Care Policy and Research.

Legoretta, Antonio P., Jeffrey H. Silber, George N. Costantino, Richard W. Kobylinski, Steven L. Zatz. 1993. "Increased Cholecystectomy Rate after the Introduction of Laparoscopic Cholecystectomy." *JAMA* 270 (12; September 22): 1469–1470.

Leichter, Howard M. 1993. "State Model: Minnesota—the Trip from Acrimony to Accommodation." *Health Affairs* 12 (2; Summer): 48–58.

Lemrow, N., D. Adams, Rosanna Coffey, and Dean Farley. 1990. *The 50 Most Frequent Diagnosis-Related Groups (DRGs), Diagnoses, and Procedures: Statistics by Hospital Size and Location.* Hospital Studies Program Research Note, no. 13. Rockville, Md.: Agency for Health Care Policy and Research.

Lessler, D. S., and A. L. Avins. 1992. "Cost, Uncertainty, and Doctors' Decisions: The Case of Thrombolytic Therapy." *Archives of Internal Medicine* 152 (8; August): 1665–1672.

Letsch, Suzanne W., Helen C. Lazenby, Katharine R. Levit, Cathy A. Cowan. 1992. "National Health Expenditures." *HCFR* 14 (2; Winter): 1–30.

Levey, Bob. 1994. "A Donation from a Satisfied Customer." *Washington Post,* January 10, final edition, sec. C, p. 12, col. 1.

Levit, Katharine R., and Cathy A. Cowan. 1991. "Business, Households, and Governments: Health Care Costs, 1990." *HCFR* 13 (2; Winter): 83–91.

Levit, Katharine R., Cathy A. Cowan, Helen C. Lazenby, Patricia A. McDonnell, Arthur L. Sensenig, Jean M. Stiller, and Darleen K. Won. 1994. "National Health Spending Trends, 1960–1993." *Health Affairs* 13 (5; Winter): 14–32.

Levit, Katharine R., Gary L. Olin, and Suzanne W. Letsch, 1992. "Americans' Health Insurance Coverage, 1980–91." *HCFR* 14 (1; Fall): 31–57.

Lewin, Lawrence S., Timothy J. Eckels, and Linda B. Miller. 1988. "Setting the Record Straight: The Provision of Uncompensated Care by Not-for-Profit Hospitals." *NEJM* 318 (18; May 5): 1212–1215.

Leyland, Jill, and Associates. 1990. *Consumer Spending Patterns in the European Community.* Special Report, no. 2044 (October). London: Business International.

Lindsay, Cotton M. 1969. "Medical Care and the Economics of Sharing." *Economica* 144 (November): 351–362.

Lomas, Jonathan, Catherine Fooks, Thomas Rice, and Roberta J. Labelle. 1989. "Paying Physicians in Canada: Minding Our Ps and Qs." *Health Affairs* 8 (1; Spring): 80–102.

Lubitz, James D., and Gerald F. Riley. 1993. "Trends in Medicare Payments in the Last Year of Life." *NEJM* 328 (15; April 15): 1092–1096.

Luft, Harold S. 1978. "How Do Health Maintenance Organizations Achieve Their Savings?" *NEJM* 298 (24; June 15): 1336–1343.

———. 1983. "The Professional Activity Study of the Commission on Hospital and Professional Activities: A User's Perspective." *Health Services Research* 18 (2, pt. 2; Summer): 349–352.

MacDonald, Maurice. 1977. *Food, Stamps, and Income Maintenance.* New York: Academic Press.

Maher, Walter B. 1990. *Rising Health Care Costs: Are They Really Making It Harder for U.S. Firms to Compete?* Joint Economic Committee. Senate Hearing 101–900 (May). Washington, D.C.: Government Printing Office.

Manga, Pranlal, and Geoffrey R. Weller. 1980. "The Failure of the Equity Objective in Health: A Comparative Analysis of Canada, Britain, and the United States." *Comparative Social Research* 3: 229–267.

Manning, Willard G., Joseph P. Newhouse, Naihua Duan, Emmett B. Keeler, Arleen Leibowitz, and M. Susan Marquis. 1987. "Health Insurance and the Demand for Medical Care: Evidence from a Randomized Experiment." *American Economic Review* 77 (June): 251–277.

Mark, Daniel B., C. David Naylor, Mark A. Hlatky, Robert M. Califf, Eric J. Topol, Christopher B. Granger, J. David Knight, Charlotte L. Nelson, Kerry L. Lee, Nancy E. Clapp-Channing, Wanda Sutherland, Louise Pilote, and Paul W. Armstrong. 1994. "Use of Medical Resources and Quality of Life after Acute Myocardial Infarction in Canada and the United States." *NEJM* 331 (17; October 27): 1130–1135.

Marmor, Theodore R. 1994. *Understanding Health Care Reform.* New Haven: Yale University Press.

Marmor, Theodore R., and James A. Morone. 1983. "The Health Programs of the Kennedy-Johnson Years: An Overview." In *Political Analysis and American Medical Care: Essays,* edited by Theodore Marmor. Cambridge: Cambridge University Press.

Marquis, M. Susan, and Joan L. Buchanan. 1994. "How Will Changes in

Health Insurance Tax Policy and Employer Health Plan Contributions Affect Access to Health Care and Health Care Costs?" *JAMA* 271 (12; March 23): 939–944.

Mashaw, Jerry L. 1993. "Taking Federalism Seriously: The Case for State-Led Health Care Reform." *Domestic Affairs* 2 (4; Winter): 1–21.

McCaughey, Elizabeth P. 1994. "No Exit." *The New Republic* 210 (February 7): 21–25.

McCord, Colin, and Harold P. Freeman. 1990. "Excess Mortality in Harlem." *NEJM* 322 (3; January 18): 173–177.

McDowell, Banks. 1989. *Deregulation and Competition in the Insurance Industry.* New York: Quorum Books.

McGlynn, Elizabeth A., C. David Naylor, Geoffrey M. Anderson, Lucian L. Leape, Rolla Edward Park, Lee H. Hilborne, Steven J. Bernstein, Bernard S. Goldman, Paul W. Armstrong, Joan W. Keesey, Laurie McDonald, S. Patricia Pinfold, Cheryl Damberg, Marjorie J. Sherwood, and Robert H. Brook. 1994. "Comparison of the Appropriateness of Coronary Angiography and Coronary Artery Bypass Surgery between Canada and New York State." *JAMA* 272 (12; September 28): 934–940.

McKenzie, Richard B. 1992. "Was It a Decade of Greed?" *Public Interest* 106 (Winter): 91–96.

McLaughlin, Catherine G., and Wendy K. Zellers. 1992. "The Shortcomings of Voluntarism in the Small-Group Insurance Market." *Health Affairs* 11 (2; Summer): 28–40.

McClellan, Mark, Barbara J. McNeil, and Joseph P. Newhouse. 1994. "Does More Intensive Treatment of Acute Myocardial Infarction in the Elderly Reduce Mortality? Analysis Using Instrumental Variables." *JAMA* 272 (11; September 21): 859–866.

Mechanic, David. 1992. "Professional Judgment and the Rationing of Medical Care." *University of Pennsylvania Law Review* 140: 1713–1754.

Miller, Jeffrey G., and Thomas E. Vollman. 1985. "The Hidden Factory." *Harvard Business Review* 63 (5; September): 142–150.

Mittelstaedt, H. Fred, and Mark J. Warshawsky. 1993. "The Impact of Liabilities for Retiree Health Benefits on Share Prices." *Journal of Risk and Insurance* 60 (March): 13–35.

Moffit, Robert Emmet. 1992. "Back to the Future: Medicare's Resurrection of the Labor Theory of Value." *Regulation* 15 (4; Fall): 54–63.

Morrissey, Michael A. 1994. *Cost Shifting in Health Care: Separating Evidence from Rhetoric.* Washington, D.C.: AEI Press.

Moser, James W., and Robert A. Musacchio. 1991. "The Costs of Medical Professional Liability in the 1980s." *Medical Practice and Management* 7 (Summer): 6–9.

Motor Vehicle Manufacturers' Association. 1992. *Motor Vehicle Facts and Figures.* Detroit: Motor Vehicle Manufacturers' Association.

Naylor, C. David, A. Andrew Hollenberg, Anne Marie Ugnat, and A. Basinski. 1990. "Coronary Thrombolysis—Clinical Guidelines and Public Policy: Results of an Ontario Practitioner Survey." *Canadian Medical Association Journal* 142 (10; May 15): 1069–1076.

Nelson, Jack. 1993. "Dole Urges GOP Support for Health Care Reform, NAFTA." *Los Angeles Times,* September 25, sec. A, p. 1, col. 3.

Neuffer, Elizabeth. 1993. "Freeze in Health Costs Is Focus of Hot Debate." *Boston Globe,* March 21, sec. A, p. 1, col. 5.

Newborns' and Mothers' Health Protection Act of 1996. Public Law: 104–204. Washington, D.C.: Government Printing Office.

Newhouse, Joseph P. 1992a. "Medical Care Costs: How Much Welfare Loss?" *Journal of Economic Perspectives* 6 (3; Summer): 3–21.

———. 1992b. "Pricing and Imperfections in the Medical Care Marketplace." In *Health Economics Worldwide,* edited by Peter Zweifel and H. E. Frech III, 3–22. Dordrecht, Netherlands: Kluwer Academic Publishers.

———. 1993a. *Free for All? Lessons from the RAND Health Insurance Experiment.* Cambridge: Harvard University Press.

———. 1993b. "An Iconoclastic View of Health Care Cost Containment." *Health Affairs* 12 (Supplement): 152–171.

———. 1994. "Health Services Research in a Post-Reform World: Presidential Address to the Association for Health Services Research." *Health Services Research* 29 (5; December): 515–521.

Newport, Frank, and Jennifer Leopard. 1991. "The Crisis in National Health Care." *Gallup Poll Monthly,* August, 4–7.

New York State Casualty Actuarial Bureau. 1995. "Private Passenger Automobile Distribution by Deductible." Fax to author, January 10.

Noether, Monica. 1986. "The Effect of Government Policy Changes on the Supply of Physicians: Expansion of a Competitive Fringe." *Journal of Law and Economics* 29 (October): 231–262.

Norton, Edward C., and Douglas O. Staiger. 1994. "How Hospital Ownership Affects Access to Care for the Uninsured." *RAND Journal of Economics* 25 (Spring): 171–185.

Office of Management and Budget (OMB). 1994. *Budget.* Washington, D.C.: Government Printing Office.

Office of Technology Assessment (OTA). 1988. *Medical Testing and Health Insurance* (August). Washington, D.C.: Government Printing Office.

———. 1991. *Medical Monitoring and Screening in the Workplace: Results of a Survey.* Background Paper OTA-BP-BA-67 (October). Washington, D.C.: Government Printing Office.

————. 1992. *Does Health Insurance Make a Difference?* Background Paper OTA-BP-H-99. (September). Washington, D.C.: Government Printing Office.

————. 1993a. *Impact of Legal Reforms on Medical Malpractice Costs* (October). Washington, D.C.: Government Printing Office.

————. 1993b. *International Health Statistics: What the Numbers Mean for the United States.* Background Paper OTA-BP-H-116 (November). Washington, D.C.: Government Printing Office.

————. 1994. *Assessing the Assumptions behind Health Reform Projections.* Washington, D.C.: Government Printing Office.

Ontario. 1993. *Ontario's Expenditure Control Plan* (April). Toronto: Publications Ontario.

Ontario Ministry of Health. 1994. *Managing Health Care Resources 1994–95: Meeting Priorities.* Toronto: Publications Ontario.

Organization for Economic Cooperation and Development (OECD). 1993a. *Economic Surveys: Canada.* Paris: OECD.

————. 1993b. *Health Care Data Base.* Paris: OECD.

Pauly, Mark V. 1971. *Medical Care at Public Expense.* New York: Praeger.

————. 1985. "What Is Adverse about Adverse Selection?" *Advances in Health Economics and Health Services Research* 6: 281–286.

————. 1986. "Taxation, Health Insurance, and Market Failure." *Journal of Economic Literature* 24 (June): 629–675.

————. 1987. "Nonprofit Firms in Medical Markets." *American Economic Review* 77 (May): 257–262.

————. 1988. "Is Medical Care Different? Old Questions, New Answers." *Journal of Health Politics, Policy, and Law* 13 (2; Summer): 227–237.

————. 1992. "The Normative and Positive Economics of Minimum Health Benefits." In *Health Economics Worldwide,* edited by Peter Zweifel and H. E. Frech III, 63–78. Dordrecht, Netherlands: Kluwer Academic Publishers.

Pauly, Mark V., Patricia Danzon, Paul J. Feldstein, and John Hoff. 1992. *Responsible National Health Insurance.* Washington, D.C.: AEI Press.

Petrie, K., K. Chamberlain, and R. Azariah. 1994. "The Psychological Impact of Hip Arthroplasty." *Australian and New Zealand Journal of Surgery* 64 (2; February): 115–117.

Phelps, Charles E. 1976. "Demand for Reimbursement Insurance." In *The Role of Health Insurance in the Health Services Sector,* edited by Richard N. Rossett. New York: NBER.

————. 1993. "The Methodologic Foundations of Studies of the Appropriateness of Medical Care." *NEJM* 329 (17; October 21): 1241–1245.

Phibbs, Ciaran S., David H. Mark, Harold S. Luft, Deborah W. Garnick, Erik

Lichtenberg, and Stephen J. McPhee. 1993. "Choice of Hospital for Delivery: A Comparison of High-Risk and Low-Risk Women." *Health Services Research* 28 (2; June): 201–222.

Physician Payment Review Commission. 1995. *Annual Report to Congress.* Washington, D.C.: Government Printing Office.

Pope, Gregory, and John Schneider. 1992. "Trends in Physician Incomes." *Health Affairs* 11 (1; Spring): 181–193.

"A Portrait of the Boss: The *Business Week* Corporate Elite." 1988. *Business Week* 3075 (October 21): 27–32.

President of the United States. 1992. *The President's Comprehensive Health Reform Program* (February 6). Washington, D.C.

Price, James, and James Mays. 1985. "Biased Selection in the Federal Employees' Health Benefit Program." *Inquiry* 22 (1; Spring): 66–77.

Priest, Dana. 1993a. "Health Care Price Caps Considered." *Washington Post,* February 14, sec. A, p. 1, col. 6.

———. 1993b. "Medical Price Caps Drafted for Clinton." *Washington Post,* March 17, sec. A, p. 1, col. 5.

Prospective Payment Assessment Commission (PROPAC). 1990. *Annual Report.* Washington, D.C.: Government Printing Office.

———. 1993. *Annual Report.* Washington, D.C.: Government Printing Office.

Puelz, Robert, and Arthur Snow. 1994. "Evidence on Adverse Selection: Equilibrium Signaling and Cross-Subsidization in the Insurance Market." *Journal of Political Economy* 102 (2; April): 236–257.

Redelmeier, Donald A., and Victor R. Fuchs. 1993. "Hospital Expenditures in the U.S. and Canada." *NEJM* 328 (11; March 18): 772–778.

Reilly, Thomas W., Steven B. Clauser, and David K. Baugh. 1990. "Trends in Medicaid Payments and Utilization, 1975–89." *HCFR* (Supplement): 15–33.

Reinhardt, Uwe. 1989. "Health Care Spending and American Competitiveness." *Health Affairs* 8 (4; Winter): 5–21.

Reischauer, Robert. 1993. *Testimony before the House Ways and Means Committee, Subcommittee on Health, Health Care Reform* (February 2), vol. 1, 149–199. Washington, D.C.: Government Printing Office.

Relman, Arnold S., and Uwe Reinhardt. 1986. "Debating For-Profit Health Care and the Ethics of Physicians." *Health Affairs* 5 (2; Summer): 5–31.

Rettig, Richard A. 1994. "Medical Innovation Fuels Cost Containment." *Health Affairs* 13 (3; Summer): 7–27.

Reynolds, Roger A., John A. Rizzo, and Martin L. Gonzalez. 1987. "The Cost of Medical Professional Liability." *JAMA* 257 (20; May 22): 2776–2781.

Rivo, Marc L., and David Satcher. 1993. "Improving Access to Health Care through Physician Workforce Reform." *JAMA* 270 (9; September 1): 1074–1078.

Roback, Gene, Lillian Randolph, Bradely Seidman, and Thomas Pasko. 1994. *Physician Characteristics and Distribution in the United States*. Chicago: AMA Department of Data Services.

Roberts, Marc J. 1986. "Economics and the Allocation of Resources to Improve Health." In *The Price of Health*, edited by George J. Agich and Charles E. Begley. Boston: D. Reidel.

Roberts, Marc J., and Alexandra T. Clyde. 1993. *Your Money or Your Life: The Health Care Crisis Explained*. New York: Doubleday.

Robinson, James C., Laura B. Gardner, Harold S. Luft. 1993. "Health Plan Switching in Anticipation of Increased Medical Care Utilization." *Medical Care* 31 (1; January): 43–51.

Robinson, John P. 1993. "As We Like It." *American Demographics* 15 (2; February): 44–48.

Roemer, Ruth, and Milton I. Roemer. 1977. *Health Manpower Policy under National Health Insurance: The Canadian Experience*. Hyattsville, Md.; Department of Health, Education, and Welfare, Bureau of Health Manpower.

Rothman, David J. 1993. "A Century of Failure: Health Care Reform in America." *Journal of Health Politics, Policy, and Law* 18 (2; Summer): 271–286.

Rouleau, Jean L., Lemuel A. Moye, Marc A. Pfeffer, J. Malcom, O. Arnold, Victoria Bernstein, Thomas Cuddy, Gilles R. Dagenais, Edward M. Geltman, Steven Goldman, David Gordon, Peggy Hamm, Marc Klein, Gervasio A. Lamas, John McCans, Patricia McEwan, Francis J. Menapace, John O. Parker, François Sestier, Bruce Sussex, and Eugene Braunwald. 1993. "A Comparison of Management Patterns after Acute Myocardial Infarction in Canada and the United States." *NEJM* 328 (11; March 18): 805–807.

Rublee, Dale A. 1989. "Medical Technology in Canada, Germany, and the United States." *Health Affairs* 8 (3; Fall): 178–181.

———. 1994. "Medical Technology in Canada, Germany, and the United States: An Update." *Health Affairs* 13 (4; Fall): 112–117.

Russ, Ray. 1993. "The Futures Look Bright." *Financial Executive* 9 (14; July/August): 45–47.

Sage, William M., Kathleen E. Hastings, and Robert A. Berenson. 1994. "Enterprise Liability for Medical Malpractice and Health Care Quality Improvement." *American Journal of Law and Medicine* 20: 1–28.

Sarkar, Debo. 1995. "The Entry of Foreign-Trained Medical Graduates." Ph.D. dissertation, Columbia University.

Schur, Claudia L., and Amy K. Taylor. 1991. "Choice of Health Insurance and the Two-Worker Household: Data Watch." *Health Affairs* 10 (1; Spring): 155–163.

Schwartz, William B. 1987. "The Inevitable Failure of Current Cost-Containment Strategies." *JAMA* 257 (2; January 9): 220–224.

———. 1994. "In the Pipeline: A Wave of Valuable Medical Technology." *Health Affairs* 13 (3; Summer): 70–79.

Sekscenski, Edward S., Stephanie Sansom, Carol Bazell, Marla E. Salmon, and Fitzhugh Mullen. 1994. "State Practice Environments and the Supply of Physician Assistants, Nurse Practitioners, and Certified Nurse-Midwives." *NEJM* 331 (19; November 10): 1266–1271.

Serbein, Oscar N., Jr. 1953. *Paying for Medical Care in the United States.* New York: Columbia University Press.

Sloan, Frank A. 1990. "Experience Rating: Does It Make Sense for Medical Malpractice Insurance?" *American Economic Review* 80 (May): 128–133.

Sloan, Frank A., Thomas J. Hoerger, Michael A. Morrissey, and Mahud Hassan. 1990. "The Demise of Hospital Philanthropy." *Economic Inquiry* 28 (October): 725–743.

Sloan, Frank A., Paula M. Mergenhagen, W. Bradley Burfield, Randall R. Bovbjerg, and Mahud Hassan. 1989. "Medical Malpractice Experience of Physicians: Predictable or Haphazard." *JAMA* 262 (23; December 15): 3291–3297.

Smith, Geoffrey N. 1986. "Follow the Money." *Forbes* 138 (1; July 14): 90–94.

Smith, Mark D., Drew E. Altman, Robert Leitman, Thomas W. Moloney, and Humphrey Taylor. 1992. "Taking the Public's Pulse on Health System Reform." *Health Affairs* 11 (2; Summer): 125–133.

Smith, Marguerite T. 1994. "The Wild New World of Health Care for Your Pet." *Money* 23 (April): 144–158.

Smith, Robert J., ed. 1993. *Medical and Healthcare Marketplace Guide,* 9th edition. Miami: International BioMed Information Service.

Social Security Administration. 1992, 1993. *Annual Statistical Supplement to the Social Security Bulletin.* Washington, D.C.: DHHS.

Somers, Herman M., and Anne R. Somers. 1961. (Reprinted 1970.) *Doctors, Patients, and Health Insurance.* Washington, D.C.: Brookings Institution.

Starr, Paul. 1982. *The Social Transformation of American Medicine.* New York: Basic Books.

————. 1994. *The Logic of Health Care Reform.* New York: Penguin Books.

————. 1995. "What Happened to Health Care Reform?" *American Prospect* 20 (Winter): 20–31.

Starr, Paul, and Walter A. Zelman. 1993. "A Bridge to Compromise: Competition under a Budget." *Health Affairs* 12 (Supplement): 7–23.

Statistics Canada. *Canada Year Book.* Various years. Ottawa: Statistics Canada.

————. 1993. *Selected Income Statistics: The Nation.* Ottawa: Statistics Canada.

Stevens, Robert, and Rosemary Stevens. 1974. *Welfare Medicine in America: A Case Study of Medicaid.* New York: Free Press.

Stevens, Rosemary. 1989. *In Sickness and in Wealth: American Hospitals in the Twentieth Century.* New York: Basic Books.

Stigler, George J. 1971. "The Theory of Economic Regulation." *Bell Journal of Economics and Management Sciences* 2 (Spring): 3–21.

Sulvetta, Margaret B. 1991. "Achieving Cost Control in the Hospital Outpatient Department." *HCFR* (Supplement): 95–106.

"A Survey of Healthcare: Surgery Needed." 1991. *Economist,* July 6, S1–S18.

Svorny, Shirley. 1992. "Should We Reconsider Licensing Physicians?" *Contemporary Policy Issues* 10 (January): 31–38.

Tallon, James R., Jr., and Lawrence D. Brown. 1994. "Health Alliances: Functions, Forms, and Federalism." In *Making Health Reform Work: The View from the States,* edited by John J. DiIullio, Jr., and Richard R. Nathan. Washington, D.C.: Brookings Institution.

Taylor, Amy, and Jessica Banthin. 1994. *Changes in Out-of-Pocket Expenditures for Personal Health Services: 1977 and 1987.* Research Findings 21. Rockville, Md.: Agency for Health Care Policy and Research.

Thaler, Richard, and H. M. Shefrin. 1981. "An Economic Theory of Self-Control." *Journal of Political Economy* 89 (2; April): 392–406.

Thorpe, Kenneth E. 1992. "Inside the Black Box of Administrative Cost." *Health Affairs* 11 (2; Summer): 41–56.

Thurow, Lester. 1984. "Learning to Say No." *NEJM* 311 (24; December 13): 1569–1572.

Tobin, James. 1970. "On Limiting the Domain of Inequality." *Journal of Law and Economics* (October): 263–277.

Van Son, Victoria. 1993. *State Fact Finder: Rankings across America.* Washington, D.C.: Congressional Quarterly.

VanTuinen, Ingrid, Phyllis McCarthy, and Sidney Wolfe. 1991. *9479 Questionable Doctors Disciplined by States or the Federal Government.* Washington, D.C.: Public Citizen Health Research Group.

Viscusi, W. Kip. 1994. "Efficacy of Labeling Foods and Pharmaceuticals." *Annual Review of Public Health* 15: 325–343.

Vladeck, Bruce. 1981. "The Market versus Regulation: The Case for Regulation." *Milbank Memorial Fund Quarterly* 59 (Spring): 209–223.

Waldo, Daniel R., Sally T. Sonnefeld, David R. McKusick, and Ross H. Arnett III. 1989. "Health Expenditures by Age Group, 1977 and 1987." *HCFR* 10 (4; Summer): 111–120.

Ward's Automotive Yearbook, 52d edition. 1990. Detroit: Ward's Communications.

Watkins, Mel, ed. 1993. *Canada.* New York: Facts on File.

Weiler, Paul C. 1991. *Medical Malpractice on Trial.* Cambridge: Harvard University Press.

Weiler, Paul C., Howard H. Hiatt, Joseph P. Newhouse, William G. Johnson, Traycr A. Brenan, and Lucian L. Leape. 1993. *A Measure of Malpractice: Medical Injury, Malpractice Litigation, and Patient Compensation.* Cambridge: Harvard University Press.

Weiner, Jonathan P., and Gregory de Lissovoy. 1993. "Razing a Tower of Babel: A Taxonomy for Managed Care and Health Insurance Plans." *Journal of Health Politics, Policy, and Law* 18 (1; Spring): 75–103.

Weisbrod, Burton A. 1991. "The Health Care Quadrilemma: An Essay on Technological Change, Insurance, Quality of Care, and Cost Containment." *Journal of Economic Literature* 29 (June): 523–552.

Weissman, Joel S., and Arnold M. Epstein. 1994. *Falling through the Safety Net.* Baltimore: Johns Hopkins University Press.

Welch, W. Pete. 1992. "Alternative Geographic Adjustments in Medicare Payment to Health Maintenance Organizations." *HCFR* 13 (3; Spring): 97–110.

Wennberg, John, and Alan Gittelsohn. 1973. "Small Area Variations in Health Care Delivery." *Science* 182 (December): 1102–1108.

White, Michelle J. 1994. "The Value of Liability in Medical Malpractice." *Health Affairs* 13 (4; Fall): 75–87.

White-Traut, R. C., and M. B. C. Goldman. 1988. "Premature Infant Massage: Is it Safe?" *Pediatric Nursing* 14 (4; July–August): 285–289.

Wilkins, Russell, Owen Adams, and Ama Brancker. 1989. "Changes in Mortality by Income in Urban Canada from 1971 to 1986." *Health Reports* 1 (2): 136–167.

Wise, J. Karl. 1984a. "Veterinary Health Care Market for Cats." *JAVMA* 184 (February 15): 481–482.

———. 1984b. "Veterinary Health Care Market for Dogs." *JAVMA* 184 (January 15): 207–208.

Wise, J. Karl, and Jih Jing Yang. 1992. "Veterinary Services Market for Companion Animals, 1992. Part II: Veterinary Service Use and Expenditures." *JAVMA* 201 (October 15): 1174–1176.

————. 1994. "Dog and Cat Veterinary Services Market, 1991–1998." *JAVMA* 204 (May 15): 1570.

Whol, Stanley. 1984. "Is Corporate Medicine Healthy for America?" *Business and Society Review* 51 (Fall): 16–20.

Wolfson, A. D., and Carolyn J. Tuohy. 1980. *Opting Out of Medicare.* Toronto: Ontario Economic Council, University of Toronto Press.

Woods, John R., Robert M. Saywell, Jr., Allen W. Nyhuis, Stephen J. Jay, Rosemary G. Lohrman, and Harold G. Halbrook. 1992. "The Learning Curve and the Cost of Heart Transplantation." *Health Services Research* 27 (2; June): 219–238.

Woolhandler, Stephanie, and David Himmelstein. 1991. "The Deteriorating Administrative Efficiency of the U.S. Health Care System." *NEJM* 324 (18; May 2): 1253–1258.

World Bank. *World Development Report.* 1993. New York: Oxford University Press.

Zelman, Walter A. 1993. "Who Should Govern the Purchasing Cooperative?" *Health Affairs* 12 (Supplement): 48–57.

Zook, Christopher J., Francis D. Moore, and Richard J. Zeckhauser. 1981. "Catastrophic Health Insurance—a Misguided Prescription?" *Public Interest,* no. 62 (Winter): 66–81.

Zwanzinger, Jack, Geoffrey M. Anderson, Susan G. Haber, Kenneth E. Thorpe, and Joseph P. Newhouse. 1993. "Comparison of Hospital Costs in California, New York, and Canada." *Health Affairs* 12 (2; Summer): 130–139.

Index

275